D1384201

Life Goes On

Journey of a Liver Transplant Recipient

BY CHRISTINE JOWETT, RN

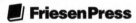 **FriesenPress**

Suite 300 - 990 Fort St
Victoria, BC, Canada, V8V 3K2
www.friesenpress.com

ISBN
978-1-4602-6709-7 (Hardcover)
978-1-4602-6710-3 (Paperback)
978-1-4602-6711-0 (eBook)

1. Biography & Autobiography, Medical

Distributed to the trade by The Ingram Book Company

Without the organ donor, there is no story, no hope, no transplant. But when there is an organ donor, life springs from death, sorrow turns to hope and a terrible loss becomes a gift.

—United Network For Organ Sharing

I dedicate this book to all those who gave the gift
of life and to all those who received that gift.

To all the doctors and nurses who cared for me.

TABLE OF CONTENTS

ACKNOWLEDGEMENTS

I would like to express my deep and sincere thanks to all the health-care professionals who took care of me, keeping me alive. Thank you to all the members of the Toronto General Hospital Transplant Team, you gave me a second chance at life. I would especially like to thank, Dr. Jordan Golubov, Dr. Eberhard Renner, Dr. Leslie Lilly, Dr. David Grant, Dr. S.S. Liau and Dr. Jane Dillon. I owe many thanks to all the transplant nurses who cared for me in the ICU, Step-Down, and the 7th floor transplant unit. I would especially like to thank my liver transplant coordinator, Jill Quance.

To all the Trillium Gift of Life transplant coordinators and staff, thank you for making my liver transplant possible.

Over the years as my disease progressed, I had the privilege of being cared for by several excellent hepatologists and gastroenterologists, Dr. Hermant Shah, Dr. Larry Lietaer, Dr. Jenny Heathcote, Dr. Jorge Marrero, Dr. Alan Buckley, Dr. John Walling, and Dr. A.P. van den Berg. Thank you for your expertise, kindness and support, allowing me to have a life while living with autoimmune hepatitis.

To my friends and co-workers at St. Mary's Hospital. Thank you for taking care of me when I was on the other side of the bed, the fundraisers, meals, and prayers. You are all truly amazing friends and colleagues.

Many thanks to Trillium Gift of Life transplant organ and tissue donation coordinator Judy Wells, and manager Colleen Colleen Shelton of the multi organ transplant unit at Toronto General Hospital for answering my many questions in order to write this book.

To, Andrea Clegg, Joanna & Ryley Mitchell, Janine Thompson, Kelly Thorman-Kleinschmidt, Shelley Armstrong, Andrea & Phil Tjart, Ken Lemon, and John Wynen, for contributing to my book and sharing your stories.

A huge thank you to my editor, Mary Ann Mazey, for your long hours, hard work, and invaluable advice.

To Lyn Ismael, thank you for taking the photographs for my book cover and author portrait. Thank you Leona Hollingsworth for providing the TGLN Human Organ cooler for the cover photograph.

There are many family members and friends that have prayed for me, sent gifts, made phone calls, and were there for me on many levels. I am blessed to have you in my life. To my husband, Kevin, thank-you for shuttling me back and forth to doctors appointments and encouraging me to write my story. I never realized how much effort goes into writing a book. This project kept me occupied and my mind busy during many months of recovery from surgery. To my children, Kyle and Sarah, thank you for all your love, hugs and kisses when I needed them the most. To my mom for always being there for me. For my dad, who made sure I never gave up. And my brothers, Andy and Bill, I know you would do whatever it takes to help out your "big sister."

During my transplant work up, when there was still hope that a living donor could save my life, my brother Bill and cousin Catherine stepped forward and were willing to donate part of their liver. I cannot thank you enough.

I hope to live a long and healthy life post transplant knowing that my guardian angel, Nana, is keeping an eye on me.

Finally, no words will ever be enough to express my deepest gratitude towards my donor and donor family for giving me the gift of life. You are the reason I am alive.

Chapter 1

BUT I'M JUST A KID

In 1987, the first anti-smoking ad aired on TV; Canada introduced the "loonie"; disposable contact lenses were invented; and the Free Trade Agreement was reached by negotiators for Canada and the United States. *The Cosby Show*, *Full House*, and *Married with Children* were popular TV shows. "Livin' on a Prayer," "La Bamba," and "(I've Had) The Time of My Life" were songs blaring from Walkman headphones. For me, 1987 was an unforgettable year because it was my last year of elementary school and the year I became sick.

In September, I was assigned to Mr. Bateman's grade eight class at Queen Elizabeth Public School (Queen E.) in my hometown of Belleville, Ontario. I was a runner, and September is the beginning of the cross-country running season. Our first meet was a five-kilometre run in Bancroft along leaf-covered dirt trails through a colourful deciduous forest. Halfway through the race, a sharp nagging pain along the right side of my abdomen was plaguing me. I attributed the pain to a side stitch and ran with my hands on my hips. The pain continued to stab me and fatigue set in, making it difficult to finish the race. There were several inviting piles of maple leaves along the trail where I wanted to lie down and nap. But my will to finish the race took over, and I placed third. Third place meant I earned three dollars. My dad had said he would give me five dollars for first place, four dollars for second place, and three dollars for third place. I didn't want to go home empty-handed!

I slept the entire hour and a half trip back to Belleville while being bumped around on the yellow school bus. When I arrived back at Queen E., my mom was in the parking lot waiting for my brother Andy and me. On our short drive home, we excitedly told Mom how we did in the race, showing her our ribbons. I told her about the side stitch and how I'd been tired during the race but had pushed myself to finish. Mom thought I might be coming down with the flu. If only it had been the flu.

Every Saturday there is a farmers' market beside city hall, with a rich variety of produce and crafts. A few weeks after the race, Mom and I perused the market for a good bargain on McIntosh apples. As we walked home, the sun shone on my freckled face and Mom commented that I "looked yellow." I will never forget this comment because it was the first time my skin took on a jaundiced appearance. My mom knew what jaundice looked like because she had been diagnosed with hepatitis B when she was seventeen-years-old, one and a half years before she became pregnant with me. She still has no idea how she contracted hepatitis.

Mom made an appointment with my pediatrician, Dr. Aileen Rackham. I was a typical child patient who only visited the doctor for routine vaccinations and injured limbs. Dr. Rackham's concerned look is forever etched in my mind. Her jaw dropped in disbelief when she saw my sick, jaundiced skin and glowing yellow eyes. I lay on the crinkly paper-covered table while Dr. Rackham examined me, gently tapping my liver, pressing my abdomen, feeling my neck, and taking my temperature and blood pressure. On the way out of the office, she handed my mom a lab requisition. At this point in my life, I had never been put through the agony of a blood draw.

At the lab, Mom accompanied me to a small private cubicle with a torture chair in which the beginning of a traumatic event in my life was about to unfold. A blue tourniquet was tightly tied around my biceps, and I made a fist while the lab tech examined my forearm for the perfect vein. I was somewhat tolerant of the procedure until the lab tech stuck the needle into my arm. I screamed so loud, other staff ran into the cubicle to see what was happening. My crying, yelling, and squirming caused the lab tech to withdraw the needle and scold me for being uncooperative.

Unfortunately, the torture didn't end there. Several staff members ganged up on me and took me to a room with an examination table. They forcefully made me lie on the table and strapped down both my arms. The lab tech managed to finish drawing blood, and all the while I screamed, cried, and kicked. I even kicked the lab tech who was trying to hold my legs still. Where was my mom during all this? Probably hiding because she was embarrassed I was her daughter. I know I would have hidden if this were my child.

Dr. Rackham reviewed the results with Mom and me. Much to our horror, the liver function tests were significantly elevated. Dr. Rackham referred me to a local gastroenterologist, Dr. Lietaer. His practice was in an office building adjacent to Belleville General Hospital. I remember riding up a few floors to his office in an old, squeaky elevator—one I was sure wasn't going to hold our weight and plummet to the ground.

I was Dr. Lietaer's only pediatric patient, but he had kids my age so he was good at talking to me on a kid level. He reviewed my lab results and said I had liver disease, probably hepatitis. He didn't go into any great detail, but he told me I had a sick liver and needed medication so it wouldn't be so sick. I remember asking him why my liver was sick. He told me my body, for some unknown reason, was trying to attack my liver because it saw it as something that didn't belong inside me—something foreign. He suggested I start with five milligrams of prednisone and undergo follow-up labs to determine if it was effective in treating my liver inflammation. This was my introduction to prednisone, and the first time I was prescribed daily medication (aside from the occasional antibiotic).

The prominent black-and-white sticker on the side of the pred-nisone bottle said *Take with food*, and Dr. Lietaer had said to take it in the morning. I didn't know why until I went to nursing school: prednisone mimics the body's natural production of corticosteroid hormones when taken early in the day. So, every day I took the small, round, white pill with breakfast. But can't it come in grape or cherry flavour? What makes it taste so bad? When it gets stuck in the mouth, it is hard to get rid of the aftertaste. I learned to chew flavourful gum or have a mint afterwards, it sort of helps.

After a month on prednisone, it was time to re-draw labs. Now I knew how horrific lab draws were and did everything in my power not to go when Mom said it was time. My first instinct was to lock myself in the bathroom. *Yes, she cannot get to me from in here.* Eventually I had to come out, but when we parked at the lab, I figured I could outsmart her. She exited the car faster than I did, providing me with an opportunity to lock myself in the car. But Mom had the keys and had had enough, and I couldn't keep my fingers pressed against the lock knob forever. Defeated again!

I wish I could remember the staff's reactions when we handed them the lab requisition. It was the same group of ladies who had held me down on our last visit. And guess what? I had to be strapped down to the examination table and restrained again. Looking back, I know I really did cause a frenzied scene of kicking, screaming, and crying at every lab draw. Mom even tried bribing me. "I'll take you to the Dairy Queen if you behave yourself." Not once did I earn a trip to the Dairy Queen.

Even to this day, I still detest lab draws. I turn my head away and shield my face with my hand. I would likely pass out or panic if I looked. After most lab draws, I treat myself. I delve into the stash of chocolate I keep at home or make a pit stop at Starbucks for a chai tea latte.

My liver function tests worsened, and my skin became more jaundiced in less than a month's time. Dr. Lietaer increased the prednisone dose to ten milligrams. He also stated, in a sarcastic kind of way, that he had some "bad" news: I was to refrain from going to school. Although he wasn't sure if I had hepatitis—and if I did, what type I had—Dr. Lietaer believed my liver disease was contagious. He also advised that my family get their hepatitis B vaccinations (hepatitis A vaccinations were not available yet). He recommended I have my own towels, utensils, and dishes, and disinfect the toilet after use. I was effectively quarantined in my bedroom most of the time to minimize contact with family and friends.

My mom was only thirty-two-years-old when I became sick. For her to manage a sick teenager was a challenge. She didn't always know the right questions to ask the doctors, and she took their advice verbatim. She also didn't know how to handle my needle phobia. But she got me to all my appointments on time. She filled my prescriptions and made sure I had enough pills for the month. She made my meals and reminded me to take my pills every breakfast. She managed to care for my brothers and dad, keep house, and work part-time sewing figure skating dresses. Like most moms, she put her family first and didn't have time for herself.

My younger brothers, Andy and Bill, did not think it was fair I got to miss school. They were also miffed because they had to receive hepatitis B vaccinations and blamed me for causing their sore arms. My brothers were seven- and ten-years-old when I first became ill, so for them, I was always their sick sister. Bill later told me that I looked great and acted fine and lived a normal life, but to him, my being sick was normal.

My pink room with rainbow-coloured wallpaper and raspberry pink carpet became my home for an extended period of time. I already had a sink in my room (Dad is a plumber by trade), which meant I could wash up without "contaminating" the main bathroom. I asked Dad for a TV in my room. Bill didn't think it was fair that I got a TV in my room and special treatment; all he got was a blanket and puke bucket when he was sick. But there wasn't much on besides kids' shows and soap operas, so I completed homework and slept most afternoons. In the evenings I watched *The Beachcombers* and *Degrassi Junior High*.

Dad always checked on me after work. Sometimes he gave me a new book to read or a new cassette tape to listen to on my Walkman. He also surprised me with a paint-by-numbers project—a woodland deer scene. I completed it, but the final result didn't resemble the box. I don't think I mixed the paint colours quite right. The trees and deer looked too orange and the birch trees were blue.

The idea of staying home in my pajamas, reading, watching TV, and sleeping sounded fantastic at first—a teenager's dream. However, after a week or two of bed rest, staying home was no longer a novelty. I missed my friends. My friend Cristy lived across the street and would bring homework. My friend Susie occasionally stopped by with homework or novels from Greenley's Bookstore, where her mom worked. I couldn't invite friends in, so we chatted through the screen door. Seeing my friends only made me miss them more.

My athletic abilities were inherited from my dad, who'd taught me how to pitch softball and play hockey on our backyard rink. A difficult thing about spending hours in my bedroom during the winter was missing out on playing hockey with dad and my brothers. I could only watch from my brothers' bedroom window. Oh, how I wanted to lace up my skates and join them.

I may have been under lock and key in my bedroom, but I did have a special friend to play with. Bandit was the black-and-white dwarf rabbit I'd joyously received from my parents on my ninth birthday. Bandit hopped around my room, and onto my bed when he wanted to visit me. He would snuggle up next to my pillow and let me pet him on his nose. I had him trained to hop down to his cage in the basement when he had to use his litter box. He and I were best friends until he passed at nine years of age, which is old for a bunny.

Occasionally, Grandma and Grandpa or Nana would visit. Nana wasn't able to visit as often because she lived and worked full-time as a nurse in Toronto, but she was an excellent pen pal, so she and I often exchanged letters. I provided health updates, and Nana would write back with words of encouragement. When they visited, they usually brought get-well gifts. I still have the Matryoshka doll from Nana. Grandma and Grandpa often brought fresh cheese curd, homemade canned raspberries, and baked goods. I didn't have a restricted diet, so I thoroughly enjoyed the treats, but more importantly I enjoyed their company. I have always had a special bond with my grandparents and nana.

Mom discussed my sick leave with the principal and with my teacher, Mr. Bateman. They believed I could pass grade eight, but I would need to keep up with homework and tests. I was always an honour roll student, so they did not foresee a problem with me grasping grade eight materials, but I would have to basically teach myself. Too bad email wasn't invented yet; communication with Mr. Bateman and my classmates would have been a whole lot easier.

I was absent from late September to late February. It was important for me to keep up with school because I wanted to graduate and attend high school with my friends and classmates. In my mind, staying behind would be like flunking a grade. It wasn't easy teaching myself, but doing homework and reading textbooks gave me something to do. If I didn't understand a concept or needed help with a subject, I phoned friends. Of course, our conversations weren't just about school. They filled me in on all the grade eight gossip, but I still felt disconnected. I wanted to laugh with friends, participate in physical education class (my favourite subject), and get dressed for school. In December, all my teachers and classmates signed a giant, pale-green construction-paper card with *Get Well Soon* written in calligraphy and a picture of a clown with tears and a sad face. I still have it.

I had to write tests under a parent's supervision. I would sit at the kitchen breakfast table, and my mom would set the oven timer. After I wrote the test, Mom placed it in a sealed envelope and Andy delivered it to Mr. Bateman. We had a courier system and it worked.

Dr. Lietaer continued to increase my prednisone dose, but my liver inflammation persisted. He had a difficult time finding the right dose for a thirteen-year-old; all his other patients were adults. In January 1988, Dr. Lietaer performed a liver biopsy to determine the cause of the liver inflammation. I was admitted to the pediatric unit at Belleville General Hospital and knew nothing about what to expect, so I was deathly frightened. As I was lying in the hospital bed watching the nurse and Dr. Lietaer prepare for the biopsy, I saw the nurse place a super-ginormous needle on the sterile white cloth on the tray table. Not surprisingly, I lost it! I darted off the bed and headed for the door, manically calling for my mom, who appeared and hugged me and told me I had to co-operate with the doctor and nurse. Now that Dr. Lietaer saw my fear of needles first-hand, he decided it was best to sedate me for the procedure.

Results from the liver biopsy indicated my liver was indeed inflamed and established that I had neither A nor B hepatitis, so I was originally diagnosed with as having "non-A non-B active hepatitis." Dr. Lietaer felt I needed a specialized doctor to take over my case, so he referred me to the Francis Family Liver Clinic at Toronto Western Hospital.

Toronto is 190 kilometers southwest of Belleville—a two-hour drive on a good day. I liked going on trips to Toronto with Mom. We didn't just go to the hospital, we also went to Tim Hortons across the street for a donuts and chocolate milk. We once visited Honest Ed's, a landmark discount store lit up in Las Vegas lights. It was fun rummaging through floors and floors of items—a kind of treasure hunt. Mom used our trips to Toronto to shop and liked to browse the Eaton's Centre with me in tow. I don't know why I was on bed rest at home but was allowed to shop in Toronto. I never questioned Mom's reasoning. I just enjoyed our Toronto field trips. When my mom couldn't drive me to my appointments in Toronto, Grandma would take me in her station wagon. Grandma has a lead foot, so I always made it to those appointments with lots of time to spare.

I first met hepatologist Dr. Heathcote in February 1988. Dr. Heathcote has since retired, but she is a world-renowned liver specialist. One of her major research interests was autoimmune hepatitis. Autoimmune hepatitis was not well researched when I first became ill. When Dr. Heathcote first reviewed my case, she too diagnosed me with non-A non-B active hepatitis. But after careful consideration, she changed my diagnosis to autoimmune hepatitis.

Autoimmune hepatitis (AIH) is a liver disease whereby the body's immune system attacks its liver cells. This immune system response causes inflammation, which is known as hepatitis. Researchers think certain bacteria, viruses, toxins, and drugs trigger an autoimmune response in people who are genetically susceptible to developing an autoimmune disorder. I often question why my body decided it didn't like my liver and treated it like a foreign object.

If not treated, AIH gets worse over time. AIH is typically chronic and can lead to cirrhosis, which is permanent scarring and hardening of the liver. Eventually, liver failure can result. AIH can occur at any age but most often starts, as it did in my case, in adolescence or young adulthood. Dr. Heathcote told me she believed the onset of puberty triggered my disease—likely the change in hormones.

Researchers believe there is a genetic factor that makes some people more susceptible to AIH. Dr. Heathcote was suspicious that my mom's medical history of hepatitis B had somehow contributed to me developing hepatitis and sent my mom to the lab. The blood test results showed that Mom had antibodies for not only hepatitis B but also hepatitis A, which was shocking as she had not previously known she had ever contracted hepatitis A. Dr. Heathcote was not able to say for sure if Mom's hepatitis somehow contributed to me acquiring AIH. What I'm afraid is that my daughter, Sarah, will develop AIH. About 70 percent of people with AIH are female. Plus, I had active AIH when I was pregnant with her, which may increase her risk of developing AIH or another autoimmune disease.

Dr. Heathcote toyed with my prednisone dose and added Imuran to the mix. Imuran is an immunosuppressant medication used in autoimmune diseases and organ transplantation. My liver responded well to the combination of prednisone and Imuran.

I loved Dr. Heathcote for her incredible knowledge and expertise, but I don't think she was used to having a young teenage patient. I wanted to know things like why my period hadn't started. I wanted to know why prednisone was causing me to gain weight. Before taking the medication, I had weighed ninety pounds. After four months on prednisone, I was almost 115 pounds. I also wanted to know how I got the disease and what was going to happen to me. I was an inquisitive kid and didn't have the Internet or access to medical journals. Dr. Heathcote was my only source for answers, and I wasn't happy when she didn't answer my questions in ways I could understand or seemed to answer my questions while addressing my mom. The other thing about being a teenage patient was that I didn't get to ask any questions alone with Dr. Heathcote. I *really* wanted to know if I could have a boyfriend and kiss him without giving him my liver disease, but I would never dare ask that with Mom next to me.

I was allowed to attend school again at the end of February 1988; autoimmune hepatitis was not contagious. Walking with my brothers to Queen E. that first day back, I thought I would never make the one and a half kilometer jaunt. I was on bed rest for so long that my legs forgot how to walk that far. I occasionally sat in a snowbank and had a rest.

It was surreal re-entering Mr. Bateman's classroom. The class welcomed me back, and my friends Cristy, Susie, and Erika had kept my seat with them in the back corner. I even managed to get in trouble (with some help) that first day by disrupting the class. The four of us laughed hysterically when Susie flung a pencil from her desk and it landed lead-first in the wall between Erika and Cristy. That pencil could have taken an eye out, but we still thought it was funny. It felt good to laugh and have fun again.

In March, I turned fourteen. The thing about being young is, I was able to regain muscle strength quickly. At this point, my liver enzymes were practically normal, and my skin returned to its regular pale, freckled colour. My autoimmune hepatitis was managed with medications. Spring meant track-and-field and softball season. I ran in every middle-distance track race on the chalk-covered natural grass track at Queen E. I earned a place on the Queen E. track team and competed at the regional track-and-field meet. For most students, it was a chance to miss a day of school and enjoy the sun while eating freezies on the bleachers. For me, it meant living with a disease that didn't interfere with life—being able to run against "healthy" teenagers and win awards.

I had attended Queen E. from kindergarten to grade eight. My grade eight graduation from Queen E. in June 1988 was a memorable celebration. When it was my turn to cross the stage and receive my diploma from Mr. Bateman, he stopped me from walking offstage and held my hand. He commended me for keeping up with schoolwork and achieving honour roll status despite my absence. As the audience enthusiastically applauded, I was humbled, but proud of myself too. There had been times when both my parents and I were concerned as to whether I would graduate with my classmates.

I attended Belleville Collegiate Institute for the first semester of grade nine, and then switched schools. Nicholson Catholic College (NCC) was my high school of choice for grades nine to thirteen. Classmates at Queen E. knew about my autoimmune hepatitis. At NCC, I had a fresh start. I was able to hide my disease and be a normal teenager.

I am pretty sure my closest friends in high school knew I had a liver disease, but we never talked about it. Boys and weekend plans were more important topics. If I needed to take my medications while at a sleepover at a friend's house, I would sneak them in the bathroom with a cupped handful of water before breakfast. All my friends had got their periods, and I felt like something was wrong with me. I didn't get mine until I was sixteen, and even then they were sporadic. I had to remind myself that my body was not the same as a normal teenager's inside.

Most boyfriends never knew I was ill because I didn't tell them. I was afraid if I did reveal my disease, they would ditch me. *Who wants to date a sick girl?* I say "most" boyfriends because my last high school boyfriend did know I had autoimmune hepatitis. I remember telling him about my disease nonchalantly, like it was no big deal. He also knew something was up because I couldn't handle much alcohol. I asked Dr. Heathcote about alcohol consumption when I was eighteen. She told me no more than two drinks per week. One drink to me was like a six-pack to friends. The liver helps to remove or process alcohol, which has always put me at a disadvantage—or an advantage depending on how you look at it.

My participation in physical activities was another way I masked my disease. I kept up with the guys in phys. ed. class and school sports. I think they secretly liked when I body-checked them during our floor hockey unit.

By being overly involved in athletic activities, I tried to prove to myself, and to my peers, that nothing was wrong with me. I joined the rowing team in grade nine and rowed for NCC during the school year and for the Quinte Rowing Club in the summer. My alarm sounded every morning at 5:30, and I would row, run, or use a rowing machine. The strenuous rowing workouts and competitive regattas were secretly physically demanding for me. My liver disease meant I had low platelets and bruised easily. Every crab caught (rowing error with the oar) bruised my legs something terrible. Carrying the boat from the boathouse to the dock left bruises on my shoulder. I was absolutely physically exhausted once I arrived home after a workout. I often struggled to make it through the day and had to succumb to napping.

Looking back, I don't know how I did it. Along with rowing, I ran cross-country and middle-distance track, was a pitcher in the local girls' softball league, and played ice hockey. I do recall sleeping through class a lot, especially right after lunch. A high school desk may be hard, uncomfortable, and smell of desk cleaner, but it makes for a good napping spot. Teachers would scold me for falling asleep in class, but I played the *I'm ill with a liver disease* card and they often let me nap. I held my honour roll status throughout high school, so teachers weren't concerned with my sleeping habits. I got the work done and assignments handed in on time. I just hope I didn't snore too much during class, or worse, drool on the desk.

I struggled with my weight during high school. Lightweight rowing required a crew average of 125 pounds, with no rower over 130 pounds. I had no problem weighing less than 125 pounds. When our crew decided to enter the flyweight division, which required a 115-pound crew average, I adopted anorexic-like eating habits and engaged in over-exercising. I ran an extra ten to fifteen kilometers per week on top of my already arduous sports schedule. I ate baby food and lots of fruits and vegetables. I could recite the calories of most foods and kept a log of calories in versus calories out. (Did you know a head of lettuce has forty-five calories?) Maintaining a low weight wasn't just to keep my body in check for rowing, it was also a means of preventing weight gain from the prednisone I took every day.

I graduated high school in June 1993. My parents attended the Athletic Awards Banquet and were proud when I received awards for Top Oarswoman and Outstanding Track Runner, as well as for winning the NCC five-kilometer road race. I was also named MVP for cross-country running. For winning a slew of rewards, I was given a school letter. Only the top male and female athletes were awarded this honour. In my high school yearbook, classmates gave me the title *Most likely to be a future Olympian*, a title I hope to fulfill when I compete in the 2016 Canadian Transplant Games in Toronto.

Graduating high school meant it was time to leave the nest and continue my studies at university. I had fallen in love with Vancouver Island—the majestic scenery, the opportunities for hiking and beachcombing, and the laid-back ambiance of island life—while visiting family there the year before, so my decision to apply to the

University of Victoria (UVic) was an easy one. My UVic acceptance letter arrived in the mail on my last day of high school.

Since both my parents worked and needed to be home to take care of my brothers, they couldn't help me move to Vancouver Island. Grandma is always up for an adventure, so she volunteered to drive me in her station wagon from Belleville to Victoria. The car was packed to the roof with all my possessions, including my mountain bike. Our eight-day road trip took us through the United States, Alberta, and finally British Columbia. We got lost in Chicago because we only had a paper map for directions. There was no navigational device back then to tell us to "turn around when possible." When we drove through British Columbia and passed a small city named Salmon Arm, I giggled at the name. How could salmon have arms?

As the ferry carried us from Vancouver to Victoria, the smell of the sea air and picturesque scenery welcomed me to my new home for the next five years.

Chapter 2

UNIVERSITY YEARS—FREEDOM 19

At nineteen-years-old, I was, like many young adults, in love with the notion of moving far away from my parents and having the freedom to do what I wanted. I felt my parents cramped my life because they strictly enforced a curfew, and Mom would wait up for me to come home after evenings out with friends, *especially* boyfriends. More than 4,600 kilometers away, Vancouver Island certainly fit the criteria. But the biggest selling feature for my move across Canada was having Nana nearby.

Nana was more like a second mom to me. When she retired from nursing, she moved from Toronto to the quaint town of Sooke on Vancouver Island to be with her only daughter, Jane, and her grand-daughter (my cousin) Catherine. I knew that by attending UVic, I would be able to see Nana more frequently and spend desired quality time with her again.

I majored in marine biology, but after spending on-the-water lab sessions puking over the edge of the boat, I changed my field of study to kinesiology. I've always had a tendency to get motion sickness. We call it the "Jowett stomach." I already had the biology prerequisites, and there was a co-op program, which meant I could alternate academic study on campus with periods of work. Only five students per year were accepted into the program, and I was lucky enough to get in.

The kinesiology co-op program was four and a half years, including the summer semesters. My co-op terms were in a variety of exercise- and recreation-related settings. I spent a term working at an athletic club as an aerobics instructor and fitness consultant. Another term was spent at a long-term-care facility as a recreation therapist organizing and leading activities for seniors. This was my introduction to chair exercises and 1940s wartime music. My favourite work term was with Sooke Parks and Recreation. I lucked out getting this job because I got paid to have fun and was able to live with Nana and Aunt Jane for the summer. I was a day camp counsellor and led children on adventures, including horseback riding and repelling.

University was a time to make new friends and learn to survive on my own. I had to learn to cook more than just Kraft Dinner for supper. Some of the friends I made in first year I still have today, thanks to email and Facebook. There was one friend in particular I met in first year that was more special than most. Kevin Edwards was a second-year physics and astronomy major. His demanding studies prevented him from partying with the rest of the students in our dorm. He hid like a hermit crab in a corner room on the second floor. I was a social kind of girl and knew everyone in our dorm—except Kevin.

One of the get-to-know-you resident games played on campus was Secret Brother–Secret Sister, similar to Secret Santa. Each participant answered a series of questions about himself or herself— where are you from; what's your major; name your hobbies, favourite music, etc.—and was given someone else's information. If you were a guy, you were assigned to be the secret brother of a girl, and vice versa. The challenge was to figure out who your secret brother or secret sister was. My secret brother wrote a message on my door, left a chocolate bar tied to my doorknob, and slipped a poem under my door. I still have this poem. It is in a frame, next to a picture of Kevin and I together, sticking our heads out of a tent:

My time is rare
In the night sky I often stare
Observations I make
Sleep I never get to take
On my floor the Engineers are lots
Rearranging the lounge more often than the artist's pots
While listening to Conservative views
I ponder the length of church pews
From where I beckon
The lake, the Salmon, the Arm is where I live, I reckon
Confused more often than not
Questions I ask a lot
This is the end of my rhyme
Hope you can find me in a short time.

My roommate tacked the poem on the bulletin board between our desks. She and I played detective and tried to solve the mystery of who my secret brother was. The lake, the Salmon, the Arm *was a little odd, is that where he's from? In the night sky I often stare? Hmmm, does he like star gazing?*

Neither of us figured out the mysterious secret brother behind the poem, but the mystery solved itself. There was a Christmas dance two weeks before the semester ended. After a few Jello shooters, my roommate and I noticed a curly-blonde-haired guy sitting at a table, drinking a beer with other guys from our dorm. I don't remember exactly how I approached him, but I do remember probing him with questions. *Who was this stranger?* The more personal information he shared, the more I thought he sounded familiar, like someone I already knew. I led him back to my dorm room, to which he eagerly followed me (probably thinking he was going to get lucky), and I pointed out the poem to him. Kevin then realized he was my secret brother.

I had a return plane ticket to Ontario for Christmas break. Kevin had been hired for his first four-month work term in Calgary at Shell and wasn't returning to campus until the summer term. There were only two weeks between our encounter and our departures for us to get to know one another. Plus it was exam time, and neither of us could afford to lose valuable study time. We spent the few precious study breaks we had going for walks and eating the occasional meal together in the cafeteria (he put ketchup on everything). I honestly thought he didn't like me more than as a friend during those two weeks together because he didn't make a move. No kiss or hand-holding, nothing! Our last night together before Christmas break, Kevin finally made a move—guess he liked me after all.

During one of our study-break treks around Ring Road, I shared with Kevin the fact that I had a liver disease. Kevin recalls I was a bit light on the details. I was still getting acquainted with him and didn't want to scare him off. Kevin later told me, "I remember you telling me it was not contagious, but I didn't quite believe you—I was a bit of a skeptic."

Prior to my moving to Victoria, Dr. Heathcote had arranged a referral to gastroenterologist Dr. Buckley. He was a very patient, kind, and caring doctor with a sense of humour, and he took the time to listen and made me feel comfortable asking questions. What I liked most about Dr. Buckley was he would personally call to remind me to get my blood tested. He knew student life was hectic and that I had a needle phobia and needed a swift kick in the butt to get myself to the lab.

The plan was for me to see Dr. Buckley for prescription renewals and lab follow-ups. Dr. Buckley kept Dr. Heathcote informed of my health status. Dr. Heathcote was responsible for all medication changes. Dr. Buckley was in no way an autoimmune hepatitis specialist; in fact, at the time, I was his only AIH patient.

I spent Christmas holidays in Belleville with my family. I had been homesick during my first semester and had missed my parents. I had often cried myself to sleep while lying in my uncomfortable wooden dorm bed listening to CDs friends had burned. When I was homesick, I called Nana and my parents. I even pleaded with my parents to let me come home and attend university at a later time. I had been looking forward to living on my own and spreading my wings. I'd thought I was strong, independent, and head smart, not the homesick type. Guess I didn't know myself as well as I thought.

When I'd left for university, I had been taller and stronger than Bill and Andy. When I returned, my brothers had grown a few inches and gained muscle. Their change in physique, and the fact they were angry with me (Bill had taken over my bedroom, but while I was home, they once again had to share a room), resulted in a few wrestling matches in which I had to succumb to defeat and even injury. For the first time in my life, the tables were turned, and I didn't look like their big sister anymore.

I flew home twice a year—for Christmas break and a couple of weeks at the end of summer—which allowed me to keep my biyearly appointments with Dr. Heathcote. My autoimmune hepatitis was well controlled, so I thought very little about my disease. There was only one medication change during my university years: the Imuran dosage doubled. Dr. Heathcote decreased my blood draw frequency to every three months. Even so, I found it difficult to visit the lab, and after each time would use my cafeteria dining card to treat myself to a peanut butter honeybun or chocolate bar.

Since I was no longer a resident of Ontario, I switched from the Ontario Health Insurance Plan (OHIP) to the Medical Service Plan of British Columbia. To be eligible for OHIP coverage, a person must reside in Ontario for 153 days in any given twelve-month period. Because I did not meet the physical-presence requirement, I was forced to change provincial health care plans. When I first moved to B.C., I had to wait three months to be eligible for health care coverage. In B.C. (and in most provinces), premiums are payable for health care coverage based on family income and size. Monthly premium rates for myself were zero dollars because I was a student and made under $22,000 per year. B.C. health care did not cover Dr. Heathcote's appointments, so I had to pay out-of-pocket and then submit the claim to B.C. health care for reimbursement.

OHIP and B.C. health care do not cover prescription medications. We had a drug plan through Dad's work, but unfortunately he was laid off and then became self-employed when I was at UVic, so we lost our drug benefits. I opted into UVic's student health plan to help cover the cost of medications. Prednisone has always been dirt-cheap, but Imuran cost one hundred dollars per month at the time, and the student plan didn't cover the full cost. I relied on monthly deposits from my dad into my chequing account to help pay for medications. I remember one instance when I attempted to withdraw money from my chequing account, and the teller informed me I had insufficient funds and was in overdraft. *Overdraft, what?* That didn't make sense because Dad had told me he'd sent Mom to the bank to deposit the medication money. It turned out my mom had used the medication money to buy Bill skates instead. I have always been good at managing money, so it was humiliating to have to borrow money from my boyfriend, Kevin.

Learning to manage my disease on my own was tricky. I was used to relying on Mom to fill prescriptions. Now I had to do that, and count pills to check that I had enough every month. I had to make sure labs were drawn in a timely manner and make my own doctor's appointments. Mom wasn't there to drive me to my appointments, so I had to bike to see Dr. Buckley on my own. It was a good thing my disease was quiet and I didn't have to pay much attention to it. There was no way I wanted my liver disease to interfere with my life. I only took my medications while alone in my dorm room. I didn't tell other students I had autoimmune hepatitis. I participated in athletic activities. I drank alcohol at resident parties.

Binge drinking was a big part of campus life. We were all of legal drinking age, and everyone drank at parties. Those who didn't have a beer or cooler in hand were geeky or weird or *something was wrong with them*. I liked to fit in and would slowly nurse a few drinks over the course of the party. That way it would look like I was drinking a lot.

During this time I was also dealing with an eating disorder, a continuation of the struggle with food and body image that had begun in high school because of my meeting weight requirements in rowing and gaining weight from prednisone. I closely counted calories and recorded my calories consumed each day. I obsessively exercised and was a fitness freak, running around Ring Road a few times a day, working out at Gordon Head Recreation Centre, and participating in athletic activity classes. I was on the lightweight junior varsity rowing team. I was in excellent physical condition but weighed a measly 115 pounds on my 169-centimeter body frame. I still thought I was overweight, so I continued to cut calories. Eating next to nothing wasn't easy because prednisone increased my appetite and gave me terrible food cravings for chocolate, red Twizzlers, and oatmeal cookie mix. *I know eating dry oatmeal-cookie mix is odd, but I still blame prednisone for causing some weird cravings*. It was a vicious cycle of undereating and overexercising. I wasn't anorexic, I told myself, because I ate junk food and binged. If I ate too much, I would make sure I ran an extra kilometre or swam a few more laps.

In my third and fourth years at university, my overexercising and stressful course load wore me down, and my body required afternoon naps. The time I dedicated to exercising was overtaken by my need to nap. I was extra vigilant in making sure I consumed less than 800 calories a day and ate healthy to control my body weight. I was taking nutrition courses as part of the requirements for my kinesiology degree, so I used my classroom knowledge and developed my own healthy eating plan. I stayed on track the best I could but occasionally allowed myself to sneak a treat. I couldn't resist picking away at chips and sugary junk during student movie nights. Plus, I didn't want other students asking why I was the only one not dipping into the chip bowl.

Looking back at my university years, I know I was fortunate I didn't endure a liver flare-up or become ill (other than an occasional cold or stomach bug). My disease burdened me with a weak immune system, but I managed to stay healthy despite living in closed quarters with germ-infested students. In the second semester of my first year, I was hanging out in a friend's room, and I remember him telling me he didn't feel well. He thought he had the flu but said he also had a stiff neck and persistent headaches. After a visit to the student health centre, the doctor diagnosed him with meningitis and sent him to the hospital.

The viral meningitis case was published in UVic's student newspaper. The name of the student was published along with a message from the student health care staff informing all students to make an appointment for their meningitis vaccination. I didn't make an appointment. Instead, I ran to the centre and demanded the vaccination instantly. I was freaked out that I would contract meningitis, which could cause a liver flare-up. I felt my neck for stiffness, checked my temperature, and tried to recall if I had had any headaches recently. I explained my liver disease to the nurse, and the fact that I'd been in the same room as the guy with meningitis. I was the first student to receive the vaccination, and thankfully I didn't contract the potentially life-threatening infection. My friend eventually recovered.

Kevin missed the whole meningitis scare because he was still on his work term in Calgary. He returned to UVic for academic study in the summer of 1994. We continued our relationship where we'd left off: getting acquainted with one another. Our studies still took priority over our relationship, so we only hung out during study breaks or on a weekend night. Otherwise, we seldom crossed paths because our lecture halls were on different sides of campus. It was difficult to expand our relationship when we rarely saw one another, so we decided to become roommates. Our parents didn't approve of this idea at first, but our arrangement worked well. We had separate rooms so we could study privately, yet we got to eat meals together, bike to school together, and occasionally go out on a date. I secretly thought that this was a brilliant way to find out if we were compatible, perhaps for future reference...

Kevin was my boyfriend throughout university. Sure, I dated other guys when he was away on his work terms, but none of them gave me the warm fuzzies like he did. Hey, I was in my early twenties with raging hormones and surrounded by a sea of good-looking, intelligent guys. How could a girl resist? I put my liver disease on the backburner and didn't think about whether or not I could transmit my disease through physical contact. I still hadn't discussed intimacy, birth control, or pregnancy with my doctors. I felt terrific and normal, and my autoimmune hepatitis was quiet. There was nothing to worry about in my mind. I did know, however, there was no way in hell I was going to get pregnant. I had big plans ahead of me, like completing my university education, getting a well-paying job, and travelling the world. As a precautionary measure, I obtained a prescription for birth-control pills from a doctor at the student health services centre. As a bonus, the student drug plan covered the cost of oral contraception.

Kevin graduated a year before me and began his career as a telescope operator at the Kitt Peak National astronomy observatory in Tucson, Arizona. After a slew of paperwork and jumping over some major hurdles, I was granted a temporary visa that allowed me to complete my final work term at the Tucson Parks and Recreation facility. Basically I taught adult fitness classes and implemented an after-school youth recreation program for underprivileged teens. The pay was poor but the living was cheap, and the sun shone every day.

In June 1998, I received my Bachelor of Science degree in kinesiology. To this day, earning my degree is one of the greatest accomplishments in my life.

Chapter 3

SOUTH OF THE BORDER

My four-month co-op work term at Tucson Parks and Recreation ended. I now held a Bachelor of Science degree in kinesiology. Kevin was still working and living in Tucson. Now where to go? What to do? I was torn because the love-struck twenty-four-year-old part of me wanted to follow my boyfriend and see where our relationship would take us; the realistic and practical part of me wanted to find a job, make money, and start living an adult life, free of essays and lab assignments. I chose to follow my heart and moved south of the border. Kevin and I rented a furnished, tiny one-bedroom apartment near the Foothills Mountains in Tucson. It was our first "home" together.

Living in the Sonoran desert in Arizona was very different from living in Canada. It was strange not to have snow in the winter and to see the sun every day. There were tiny geckos everywhere. Sometimes I found those creepy critters in my shoes! One time I found a scorpion in my running shoe. After that, I always checked my shoes before slipping them on. When Kevin and I went hiking or mountain biking along the rugged, cactus-laden trails, we had to be extra vigilant about watching out for rattlesnakes. On more than one occasion, we saw a rattlesnake and had to take a detour off the trail. We weren't accustomed to fifteen-foot-tall saguaro cacti or prickly pear cacti either. They were so old and beautiful, yet very prickly. I learned just how prickly when I tripped and ended up with a palmful of needles.

I obtained a non-immigrant TN visa and could temporarily work in the United States under the title "recreation therapist." I managed to find employment as a fitness instructor at the Tucson Medical Centre's FitCenter. FitCenter was a medical fitness facility with a nice, warm rehabilitation pool, a cardiac rehab area, and a fitness studio. I truly loved my first "real" job. Being the exercise guru I am, this job was perfect. I got paid to exercise. I taught an average of six, one-hour classes a day. Halfway through each day, I took a sleep break. My co-workers were used to finding me curled up in the staff room on the floor with my blanket and pillow. One of the fitness instructors put a comic on my desk of a kitten sleeping, with the caption, "When In Doubt…Take A Nap."

Kevin worked an unusual schedule of seven nights on and seven nights off. Because the Kitt Peak observatory was way out in the Sonoran desert, ninety kilometers southwest of Tucson, he spent his seven nights on the mountain. Once in a while I would visit Kevin, but I didn't own a car, so trips up the mountain were infrequent. One time I got some crazy, hare-brained idea to cycle to the observatory. Picture this: I cycled ninety kilometers in the hot desert heat, with the last stretch of the jaunt up a fifteen-kilometer switchback mountain road, to an altitude of 2,097 meters. *What was I thinking? I know, I was following my heart.* Then the next day I got to take that dangerously steep road back down the mountain. By the time I made it to the bottom, the brake pads on my bicycle were worn down to nubbins.

My family was way up in Canada, and Kevin was working on a mountaintop half the time, so this was my first time really being alone. I kind of liked all the freedom and adventures I had—some good, some not so good. Cycling only got me so far and sometimes led to heat exhaustion. I couldn't afford a car, so I spent 800 dollars on a motorcycle and got what I paid for. That 1989 Suzuki GS500 left me stranded many times. I didn't have the money for repairs and eventually learned how to monkey around with the choke and battery to get it started. Riding a motorcycle was a blast and I felt like a cool biker chick. I'm sure I didn't fit the part, though, because I often rode wearing Birkenstocks.

Unreliable as it was, the motorcycle allowed me to get a second job at Sierra Tucson, a well-known addictions treatment center, forty kilometers away from Tucson. And it allowed me to go on many hiking adventures and visit Kevin up the mountain…until the day it caught on fire when I was taking Kevin to work on the back of it. I replaced that piece of junk with a 1996 250cc Honda.

It became a little lonely spending most of my time without Kevin. I decided I needed a friend, so I adopted a grey-and-white mini lop rabbit. I named her Twister because she liked to kick her heels up and twist around the house. Once when I took her out for a hop on the grass in front of our apartment at dusk, I noticed something moving beside her. I did a double take and realized it was a tarantula—one that belonged in a cage at the desert museum. I quickly rescued Twister and took her inside. A few days later I had another tarantula encounter. I just *knew* it was the same one. It was in front of the apartment door and I needed to bring my groceries inside. I threw cans of Chef Boyardee from my grocery bag at it until it scurried away.

I was learning to live on my own and learning to manage the little money I had. Kevin carried health care benefits, but we weren't married so I didn't qualify for coverage under his plan. If I had been a full-time employee at FitCenter, I could have paid into a drug plan and received medical and drug coverage through the center's health insurance company. However, I was considered a three-quarters-time employee. What I have learned is that many American employers do not want to pay medical benefits, so they give their employees only part-time work, or a few hours short of full-time work, like in my situation.

I no longer qualified for British Columbia health care because I was no longer considered a resident of British Columbia. I no longer qualified for traveller's insurance, either, because I had lived outside of Canada for more than six months and was no longer considered a "traveller." So, like many American citizens, I lived in America without health care.

I knew I should find a doctor to follow my condition and prescribe my medications, but I couldn't afford one. I got to see first-hand what it's like to be a poor American and not be able to afford health care. I looked into the cost to get a blood test—one hundred dollars for a basic chemistry panel and liver enzymes. *One hundred dollars!* I could have bought groceries for a month with that. I tried to find a gastroenterologist to follow me. After learning one doctor's visit was going to cost me an additional fifty to one hundred dollars per visit, depending on how much time the doctor spent with me, I decided that wasn't feasible and never settled on a doctor. I called Dr. Buckley and asked him if he could provide me with prescriptions. Being the personable and understanding doctor he is, he made me a deal. He would renew my prescriptions so long as I did a blood test each time I went back to Canada to visit family. It was a deal, and one I could afford.

There was one problem with this plan, however. Dr. Buckley could only write prescriptions in Canada, so I had to fill those prescriptions at a Canadian pharmacy. I had Nana pick up my prescriptions and mail them to me. She wrote *Prescription Medications* on the customs form and enclosed the receipts. I could barely afford my ten milligrams of prednisone and 150 milligrams of Imuran daily, but I needed them to keep me alive. Every month I sent Nana a cheque for 120 dollars to pay for my medications and to cover the cost of postage.

Things might have been stable with my liver disease, but stupid, stupid me, I had to find out the implications of not having health care in the United States. I was watching a movie late one evening alone in our apartment. I plugged in the kettle to make a cup of tea. When it was ready, I unplugged it, lifted it off the counter, and accidentally dropped the entire kettle of boiling water all over my right foot. I cursed and screamed and danced in agony around the kitchen. I climbed onto the counter and placed my foot under cool running water. The pain was horrendous. It was the worst pain I have ever experienced, hands down, and I still say this after birthing two kids and having a liver transplant.

Then I did something else that was dumb. I drove myself to the hospital in Kevin's truck. I had to drive using my left foot on both the gas and brake. I don't remember much of the drive, but I do know that when I got to the ER, I couldn't stop wailing and carrying on, and the nurse took me in right away. *Likely to stop me from scaring patients in the waiting room.*

My right foot sustained second-degree burns over the entire surface, including my toes and parts of my ankle. The burn was so nasty that the skin had peeled off and was dark brown, like the flesh was cooked. I could even see my tendons in a couple of places. The nurse started an IV and gave me morphine for the pain. An ER doctor debrided (removed the damaged tissue from) my foot, a process that wasn't as bad as I had imagined, thanks to my morphine-induced haze. He applied a silver-zinc sulfadiazine cream over my foot and then covered it with a light gauze dressing. He also lent me crutches because walking was excruciatingly painful.

I had to complete paperwork before being discharged. The clerk asked for my health insurance card, but I didn't have one to present to her. The clerk told me they would send me a bill. *How much was this accident going to cost me?* I've heard ER visits can be costly and require some people to mortgage their house just to make the payments.

The bill came in the mail a few weeks later. I set the envelope on the kitchen table, afraid of what the damage was going to be. I knew I had to open it eventually, and when I did, it said 5,000 dollars. *What the . . . !?!* Where was I going to come up with 5,000 dollars?

Maybe I could talk sweetly to the clerk and beg her to reduce the charges. Yes, that is what I would do.

Miraculously, my bill was reduced down to 350 dollars. How did I manage this? I worked at FitCenter, which is operated by the Tucson Medical Center. Because I worked for the same hospital where I was treated, they deducted the 350 dollars from my pay cheque and ate the cost for the rest of my bill. Also, I spoke to the ER clerk, the ER doctor who treated me, and a couple of accommodating ladies in the billing department. Wow, I was lucky!

Our time in Tucson was short-lived. Kevin was laid off from Kitt Peak after two years' employment. A few months later, I was also laid off. The Tucson Medical Center was unable to fund the cost of operating FitCenter. We were both forced to leave Tucson to look for other employment. Kevin took a full-time engineering physicist position at the Cyclotron Laboratory at Michigan State University in Lansing. I had secured a part-time job in Charlotte, Michigan, at the Hayes Green Beach Memorial Hospital, as a wellness instructor. It was another job teaching fitness classes and conducting personal training sessions. It too paid a piddling sum, and now I had to drive thirty minutes both directions and deal with winter driving.

We loaded our few belongings into Kevin's blue Chevy S10 pickup truck and drove for five days and across eight states to Lansing, Michigan. We made a road trip out of our move. We even stopped in Memphis to look for Elvis. Twister bunny joined us on our adventure. I could see the tourists pointing and laughing at me as I "walked" my pet rabbit on her leash at rest stops.

We made it to Lansing on December 31, 1999. A new decade and a new chapter in our lives were about to begin.

Chapter 4

BORN IN THE U.S.A.

We lived in Lansing, Michigan, from December 1999 to December 2005, exactly six years. It wasn't the prettiest place to live. There were dilapidated houses in many low-income neighbourhoods. Freeways and unkempt roads intersected the city, with box stores and abandoned industrial buildings interspersed throughout. Local news stories were often about dead bodies, shootings, and missing persons. *I'm not leaving a good impression, am I?*

The one good thing about living in Lansing was the drive to Belleville was only six hours on a good day—when border-crossing officials didn't interrogate me. This made it possible to visit family and friends more frequently. I often took advantage of long weekends and would spend holidays in Belleville. I sold my motorcycle before our move to Lansing and bought a Honda civic hatchback. It wasn't as much fun to drive, but it was better suited for wintertime in Michigan.

We rented a one-bedroom apartment close to work so we could bike (when it wasn't snowing). We only lived there for two years because some crazy things happened in that apartment complex. The thing that finalized our decision to move was learning a dead body was found in the apartment above ours. Police interviewed us to find out if we had heard any foul play or a gunshot—we hadn't. We had smelled something strange, like rotting garbage, in the hallway, but we never suspected what it was.

We bought our first house, a 1947 smoky blue bungalow in a safe, family-friendly neighbourhood. It cost us 95,000 dollars. In Canada, that would have been a mortgage down payment. The house didn't need any fixing up and had a lot of charm and character, including a laundry chute from the bathroom to the basement. The house was even close enough for both of us to continue biking to work.

Kevin and I were heavily into mountain bike racing. Or maybe I should rephrase that: Kevin was a mountain biking guru and I tagged along. We joined the Michigan Mountain Bike Association and spent our weekends racing. Kevin and I both have a competitive streak and love the outdoors, so racing suited our personalities. We participated in the Iceman Cometh Challenge mountain bike race for several years, a forty-seven-kilometer bike race in November that follows rugged trails along fields and through wooded areas.

I also played on the Capital Crush women's recreational ice hockey team. We played in some pretty seedy areas in the Detroit area, where we made sure we locked our doors and took all our belongings into the arena with us. One of our teammates kept a gun in her glove compartment. I wouldn't have been surprised if women in our league kept a gun in their hockey bag next to their beer.

Living in Michigan was a time of growing up and settling down. Sure, I still had fun and went on some crazy adventures, but I was now in my late twenties. It was time to buy a house (check), get married, and have a family. In the traditional scheme of things, that is how I saw "growing up and settling down." I did, however, also continue to get this restless itch every few years where I needed to make a big move or a life-altering change.

It took several years to convince Kevin to marry me and for the right time to present itself. We officially tied the knot on a beautiful August day in 2000 at the River Inn, in Corbyville, Ontario (a hamlet near Belleville), in an outdoor ceremony and surrounded by our family and closest friends. Mom made my wedding dress and the bridesmaid dresses, and Kevin and I grew sunflowers in my grandparents' garden that we used to decorate the venue. Kevin's parents supplied wine from British Columbia. Every girl dreams of her wedding day, and I have to say, cheesy as it sounds, that ours was a dream come true because I finally married my best friend.

Another part of growing up was that it was time to establish a career. What could I do with a kinesiology degree? I didn't have the money or desire to continue on in school. I had to carefully choose where I applied because not all employers were willing to hire a Canadian with a temporary TN visa. I wanted to do something other than teach fitness classes and found work as a physical therapy assistant at Tri-Country Rehab. I should have been given the title "massage therapist" because I predominantly massaged clients' hips, knees, backs, necks—really any ailing body part. I also did pool therapy with special needs children, and children who were involved in accidents. This part of the job was fun, but I left Tri-County Rehab after a year, in April 2001. I had a university degree and was only making eleven dollars and fourteen cents per hour. *How did people live off the five dollar and fifteen cents per hour minimum wage?* Thankfully, living in Lansing was cheap and Kevin and I could split our mortgage payments, or we would have been stuck living in the "dead-body apartment building."

Job hunting on the Web, I came across a cardiovascular technician job at Sparrow Hospital's Heart and Vascular Center. I did not meet most of the job requirements—ability to read EKGs, ability to start IVs, CCT certificate (whatever that was). But I did meet *one* requirement: I had a degree in an exercise science–related field. I figured all the rest of the qualifications, I could learn with on-the-job training. So I applied. Go figure, I lucked out and was offered full-time employment. The starting wage was eighteen dollars and twenty-five cents per hour and included full medical and dental benefits. I had landed my dream job!

My new job required me to dress like a nurse in hospital scrubs, wear a hospital badge, and don a stethoscope around my neck. I truly felt professional in my uniform. All my other jobs had required me to wear sports attire. I didn't have the money to buy scrubs, so Mom took me to Fabricland and helped me sew some. I mostly chose heart-patterned material to coordinate my uniform with my job in the Heart and Vascular Center. *Good thing I didn't work in a gastrointestinal unit. I don't think material comes in stomach and liver patterns.*

I was very intimidated my first weeks on the job. I had no idea how to read an EKG. The wavy lines with spikes and dips were like reading a foreign language. Nothing made sense. However, I had the most wonderful preceptor nurses, and they taught me well. I also studied EKG books, which I borrowed from the hospital library. I attended lunch-and-learn sessions on EKG interpretation. In due time, I became proficient at reading EKGs and EKG tracings, which to this day are still part of my job.

I also had to learn how to start intravenous lines. I knew I'd signed up to do this job, but with such a horrid fear of needles, this was a serious problem for me. How was I going to jab a very large (in my opinion), very sharp needle into a patient's vein? *What if I start an IV and I panic and faint . . . that won't be so good for the patient . . .* So how did I overcome my needle phobia? Hypnotism. I was not a big believer in hypnosis, but what other choices did I have? I couldn't tell my supervisor that I was afraid of needles. Patients needed IVs started so they could receive medications or a radioactive tracer during their stress test. *There was no getting out of this!*

A hypnotist sat me across from him in a quiet, dim room, in a comfy chair, with my eyes closed. He had me practise many deep-breathing exercises. I was half-expecting him to swing a pendulum back and forth and say, "You're getting sleeping now." Instead, he used his soothing voice and the relaxing atmosphere to put me into a hypnotic state; I felt like I was taking a nap. Then he gave me a needle like the IV needle I would be using at work, and an orange.

Even the thought of sticking an orange was petrifying. I practised the deep-breathing exercise while piercing the orange with the needle. *Breathe in, one, two, three . . . breathe out, one, two, three.* This wasn't so bad, but then again, it was an orange, not a person. *A person will have blood and veins and will scream at me if I miss.*

Surprisingly, I managed to become proficient at starting IVs on people. I don't know if the breathing exercises and hypnosis helped me conquer my fear of needles, or if it was the power of mind over matter. I still get anxious, my mouth gets dry, and I feel warm and queasy whenever I'm on the receiving end of needles, though.

Now I had to complete the Certified Cardiographic Technician (CCT) certification, which required me to take a three-hour exam testing my knowledge on reading EKGs, performing stress tests, reading holter monitors, and knowing how to handle cardiovascular emergencies, such as a heart attack. I have always been a good test writer, so the certification was easy to obtain. Still, I have kept it valid all these years because I don't want to write the test again.

I truly loved my job, and there were times when I saw why it required me to respond to emergency situations. On the first of these occasions, a forty-eight-year-old man was running on the treadmill during his stress test when his heart rhythm changed from normal sinus to a life-threatening ventricular fibrillation rhythm. He was running and boom . . . he fell onto the treadmill and went flying off the back of it. *Like something you would see in a cartoon.* I quickly pushed the emergency stop button on the treadmill, and the two doctors in the room started CPR. I pushed the emergency code button to alert staff to the cardiac arrest in the stress room. The patient was successfully resuscitated and received a stent in his left main coronary artery (commonly called the "widow-maker," this is the artery in the heart that will cause a massive heart attack if blocked, affecting middle-aged men more than anyone else). I can still see the image in my mind of the man lying on the end of the treadmill, unresponsive, his face white as a ghost and chewed up from the treadmill belt.

I worked as a cardiovascular tech until the end of 2005. Like so many people, I took some time, and a few jobs, to find my niche in the working world. While working at Sparrow Hospital, I was presented with an amazing opportunity I could not pass up. The hospital had a nursing shortage, so Sparrow Hospital offered a nurse recruitment program. For anyone interested in becoming a nurse, the hospital would provide tuition reimbursement for courses and labs. There were some stipulations to the program, including that each registered nurse had to commit to two years full-time or part-time employment at Sparrow Hospital after graduation. I didn't have the money to pay for tuition, but this RN incentive program solved my problem, and I was up for the challenge.

Lansing Community College only accepted about sixty students each year into its nursing program and used a points-based system to pick the top applicants. I was given points for having a Bachelor of Science in kinesiology and for current employment in the medical field. A certain number of points were awarded for each high school GPA. It was a nerve-wracking wait to find out if I was accepted into the program, as I knew it was competitive. Students from all over Michigan applied. I was very fortunate and truly excited when I received my acceptance letter. *Whoo-hoo, more school . . . just what I was hoping for.*

I graduated with a nursing degree in May 2005. I only attended nursing school for two years. Nurses are now required to attend a four- or five-year nursing program and attain a Bachelor of Science degree in nursing. I did an accelerated second-degree program because I had completed many of the program requirements as part of my kinesiology degree. The courses I had to complete were the nursing-based lectures, labs, and practicums in hospitals and clinics—all the interesting components. In labs we practised injections on one another. I was now okay with sticking my class-mates, but in no way was I able to offer my arm to a student nurse. Knowing she had only practised on an orange wasn't going to cut it. I had to play the hepatitis card and told my lab instructor that it wasn't a good idea to have other students exposed to my blood. I was also comfortable enough with my disease, at this point in life, to share information about my autoimmune hepatitis during class discussions on gastrointestinal diseases and conditions.

At the time of my graduation, there were no nursing vacancies in the Heart and Vascular Center at Sparrow Hospital, but I found an opening for a full-time night position as a registered nurse in the mother-baby department. The job description stated that new graduates were welcome to apply. I had liked my labour and delivery rotation in nursing school, so I applied for the job. I had next to no experience with newborns or pregnant women, but I still landed the job. I thought my job in cardiology was my dream job until I started working in mother-baby. I didn't care for nights, but I absolutely loved giving newborns their first baths and dressing them in the adorable outfits their parents provided, and rocking them and snuggling with them. When they cried, I got to hand them back to their mothers for feeding. The new moms were fun to teach; many had no idea how to change a diaper or how to console their screaming baby. I also learned how to teach new mothers to breastfeed. I didn't have any experience with this when I first started, so I learned from the pros—the older, more experienced nurses who had been there and done that with their own children.

Working as a full-time RN meant I carried health care benefits. However, I relinquished them and received extra pay in lieu of benefits because after Kevin and I got married, I qualified for spousal benefits through his work. I was no longer a "poor American" having to scrimp and scrounge to pay medical bills. I didn't have to use the ER in place of a family doctor, like many Americans do. I was the proud owner of a BlueCross BlueShield health care card.

With my new spousal coverage, I'd found a family doctor, and she referred me to Dr. Walling at the Michigan Gastroenterology Institute. Before my initial consult with Dr. Walling, I had Dr. Buckley and Dr. Heathcote fax my medical records to him. I didn't want to start over from square one and have to explain the history of my disease and current treatment plan. Dr. Walling reviewed my records and read that my last liver biopsy was back in January 1988, when I was first diagnosed with autoimmune hepatitis. His plan was to re-biopsy me. *This wasn't what I'd had in mind.* Dr. Walling told me he needed to re-biopsy my liver to find out how active my disease was and if I had cirrhosis. I was reluctant to have another biopsy because I could still remember the size and feeling of the needle embedded deep into my liver, snipping a piece of tissue out during my first biopsy at thirteen (although I'd received conscious sedation, I had still been partially aware of what was going on). After much discussion, I agreed.

Dr. Walling numbed my abdomen "a little" with some local lido-caine injections but refused to sedate me, and I had to suffer through the biopsy and an extremely painful recovery period afterwards. The biopsy results indicated that I still had a normal synthetic liver func-tion, with mildly active, chronic hepatitis, and large areas of scarring and collapse. It was the first time I learned I had liver cirrhosis, the irreversible scarring of the liver. My healthy liver tissue was now scarred for life. My liver was never going to be able to recover. It was only going to get worse. Medications would buy me time—but how much?

Dr. Walling referred me to a liver specialist, Dr. Jorge Marrero, at the University of Michigan Medical Center in Ann Arbor. Dr. Marrero specialized in gastroenterology and transplant hepatology. I was humbled to be referred to him; he was like a walking medical encyclopedia. I liked that he took the time to explain everything in simple terms and always asked for my opinion when changing medications or scheduling a procedure. During my first appoint-ment with him in October 2001, Dr. Marrero spoke to me about liver transplantation. It was the first time I heard a doctor say "liver transplantation." To me, it was like hearing I had cancer. I sobbed on Kevin's shoulder. I didn't know anything about liver transplanta-tion at this point. Nothing. I had never given any thought to having a new liver. I was never sick enough before.

Although I felt well, my recent lab results indicated that I was having a liver flare-up. My liver enzyme values were much too high, so Dr. Marrero increased my prednisone dosage and suggested I start taking Actonel once a week to help increase my bone density. He figured that due to years of prednisone use, I likely had a low bone density. With all the mountain bike racing and ice hockey I participated in, I was susceptible to bone breakage.

At the time of this appointment, Kevin and I did not want children—yet. We were twenty-seven-years-old, had only been married for a year, and were having too much fun. Since kids weren't in our plans, I was taking birth control. Dr. Marrero was in favour of me holding off on having kids, as well, since my liver enzymes were not normal.

On my next appointment with Dr. Marrero, he decided to add the anti-rejection drug mycophenolate mofetil (CellCept) to the mix because my liver enzymes were still elevated despite taking twenty-five milligrams of prednisone and 150 milligrams of Imuran daily. I also began to experience pruritus, whereby my palms and bottoms of my feet would excessively itch. I had scratched sections of skin off my palms and feet as I reflexively scratched day and night. I learned that pruritus is one of the annoying symptoms associated with liver and biliary disease. The itching is believed to be the result of the accumulation of bile acids in the skin due to the inability of the liver or bile ducts to eliminate bile acids normally. Dr. Marrero prescribed cholestyramine (Questran), an orange-flavoured powder that I would mix in water and drink three times a day. This drug, along with layers of hydrocortisone applied to my skin, gave me itch relief.

Between October 2001 and March 2004, I endured multiple AIH flare-ups. Dr. Marrero continued to toy with my medications, including adding the anti-rejection drug tacrolimus (Prograf). I hated Prograf because I had to get my blood tested more frequently to ensure the level of it in my blood was therapeutic. My liver enzymes were up and down and my disease was not very stable. I was subjected to my first gastroscopy—not a pleasant procedure,

I must say. *Let's see . . . stick a long, narrow tube down the throat, into the stomach, and make the patient gag.* I was sedated during the gastroscopy, so I don't remember much about the actual procedure. What I do remember is the unpleasant vomiting afterwards and for the remainder of the day. The gastroscopy showed a few varices— enlarged blood vessels—in my esophagus. Dr. Marrero started me on the medication Nexium ("the purple pill"), which reduces stomach acid and lessens the risk of developing stomach ulcers. Nexium really helped me out. I no longer had heartburn, and subsequent gastroscopies showed my varices had healed.

When I turned twenty- nine, Kevin and I discussed having a family. Or, as Kevin would say, my maternal urges kicked in. Before I could attempt to get pregnant, I was weaned off the two immuno-suppressants, CellCept and Prograf, because there was not enough safety data on the adverse effects to the fetus. I also discontinued Actonel and Nexium, because they weren't life-sustaining medications and I could not find concrete safety data regarding their effects on a fetus or newborn. I was concerned about getting pregnant. Would my meds harm my unborn child? Would my disease get worse or be passed on to my child? So many worries! I spent hours at the Sparrow Hospital library searching for medical articles on autoimmune hepatitis and pregnancy. Two case studies peaked my interest when I read that some women experience a remission of AIH during pregnancy.

The interesting thing about my pregnancy was, I didn't know I was pregnant. I was one of those women who didn't gain weight, was spotting (like a monthly cycle), and didn't feel any fetal movements. I discovered I was pregnant in a funny sort of way. I'd been taken off most of my meds, and my disease was managed with ten milligrams of prednisone and 150 milligrams of Imuran. Dr. Marrero was afraid I would endure another liver flare-up, so he didn't want me taking too long to get pregnant. He had me visit a fertility doctor to perhaps "speed up" the process. He also informed me that women with liver disease often have difficulty getting pregnant and carrying a fetus full term. With these concerns in mind, one morning I visited the fertility clinic at Sparrow Hospital. When I went back to the clinic after work, the nurse handed me a copy of the results of my urine test and giggled as she told me, "You are already pregnant." I screamed and jumped up and down like I won the lottery. The fertility doctor examined my uterus. He figured I was about fifteen weeks along. *Was this doctor for real?* The whole first trimester had passed and I'd missed it. I skipped the first three months in the *What to Expect When You're Expecting* book and started at month four.

I told Kevin the news right away: we were going to be parents, yeah! But I waited to tell our parents they would be expecting their first grandchild. You see, I had planned to play in a hockey tournament in Toronto the following weekend, and I was bound and determined to continue with my plans. That is what I did—I played in a women's ice hockey tournament at sixteen weeks pregnant. My mom and brother Andy watched some of my games, and after the last game, Mom said I looked a little sluggish on the ice. *Okay, here goes . . .* "That is because I'm pregnant." Mom and Andy were *very* surprised, and I was happy the tournament was over because I don't think Mom would have let me back on the ice.

Dr. Marrero kept a close eye on my liver enzymes in the second and third trimesters. Labs were drawn biweekly. I was also under the care of a high-risk pregnancy obstetrician, Dr. Steven Roth, at the Sparrow Hospital Perinatal Center. I knew Dr. Roth because I'd done a clinical rotation with him in my student nursing days. I also worked with him in the mother-baby unit. It was a little uncomfortable working with a doctor who knew me on a very personal level. Nevertheless, I liked Dr. Roth as both my doctor and a co-worker.

Being high-risk meant I had fetal ultrasounds every month. I didn't want to know the baby's sex, but I could read ultrasounds and knew as soon as the ultrasound tech performed my twenty-week scan that we were having a boy. Boy or girl, it didn't matter. What mattered was the baby's health. With that ultrasound, my expected due date was December 26—a Christmas baby. My son was healthy and continued to develop right on target for his gestational age, but with every ultrasound, I worried that my medications would affect his growth and development.

During my pregnancy, I went into remission with my disease, just like the women in the case studies I'd read. Dr. Marrero told me that the increase in estrogen and progesterone hormones, and the presence of the hormone hCG (Human Chorionic Gonadotropin) during pregnancy, likely caused some women to experience remission with their disease. I liked being pregnant because I had an excessive amount of energy and exercised every day. I didn't need to nap all the time. I couldn't sit still and always had to be doing something.

With all my extra pent-up pregnancy energy, I decided to challenge myself and participate in the five-day, 565-kilometer DALMAC bike tour from Lansing to Mackinaw City. I was five months pregnant at the time, so I had a bit of a baby bump that made it a little uncomfortable to lean forward onto my handlebars. I had to remind myself to keep my posture upright most of the ride. The most challenging thing about the DALMAC was having to pee every few kilometers. I was at that point in my pregnancy where my bladder felt like it was about to explode. There weren't any port-a-potties or public bathrooms en route, so I did what any pregnant woman would do in my situation: I squatted in cornfields or hid behind bushes. I was annoying Kevin, who had to wait for me alongside the road. What was also challenging about this ride was that I had worked a twelve-hour midnight shift the night before beginning it; my balance was a little off because I was tired, and I sometimes dozed off while cycling. The bike ride seemed to lull the baby to sleep, too, because he was a very active little fellow, but I never felt him kick while I pedalled.

At eighteen weeks I had to take the glucose tolerance test to screen for gestational diabetes. The test checks how well the body regulates its sugar levels during pregnancy. My long-time prednisone usage increased my risk of developing gestational diabetes.

Unfortunately, I failed the test miserably, meaning my pancreas did not produce enough insulin quickly enough to properly regulate my blood sugar. When I failed the test again at twenty-four weeks, I was diagnosed with gestational diabetes.

Having gestational diabetes meant I had to prick my finger four times a day—after every meal and at bedtime. The glucometer Dr. Roth gave me recorded each blood sugar measurement. I had to visit the perinatal clinic weekly to download the results. On more than one occasion, Dr. Roth lectured me on eating too many carbohydrates. It was summer and it was raspberry season. "Blame the raspberries," I would tell him. I couldn't resist my favourite food. Then came Halloween, and it was all I could do not to eat the leftover candy I'd bought for our trick-or-treaters. Then there were the Thanksgiving desserts I had to skip. And then, of course, in December I had to avoid strolling down the Christmas candy aisles in stores. Candy canes and hot chocolate were not part of my diabetic diet. If my blood sugar was not well controlled, I would have to give myself insulin injections. That was incentive enough not to eat sweets. I had no choice but to stick to a low-carb diet. Chicken wings were low carb, so I feasted on Hooters chicken wings—my pregnancy craving. I knew I was eating too many wings because the Hooters girls knew me by name and would ask me about my pregnancy progress. They even snuck a few extra wings into my orders.

Working with newborns and new moms in the mother-baby unit made me wish my pregnancy would speed along so I too could hold and snuggle my sweet newborn baby.

Kyle Robert Edwards was born two weeks before his due date, just in time to celebrate his first Christmas—a perfectly healthy six-pound, four-ounce baby boy. I actually had an easy delivery au naturel. I'd been in denial that I was actually in labour and didn't go to the hospital until my contractions were five minutes apart, so there had been no time for an epidural. Plus, there was no way I would have let an anesthesiologist touch my back with a needle that looked ten feet long.

I had a liver flare-up immediately after delivery. The labour and delivery nurses (my co-workers) were the first to notice that my skin and eyes were a bright yellow colour. Not only did I become jaundiced, I also became nauseous and itchy. I was back at it, excessively scratching my skin to the point I drew blood. Dr. Roth ordered blood work, and sure enough, my liver enzymes were way out of whack—three times their normal values. My autoimmune hepatitis flare-up was controlled with IV Solu-Medrol (liquid prednisone). I was given sixty milligrams per day of oral prednisone after I was discharged home, and over the course of the next five months, Dr. Marrero had me taper it back down to ten milligrams. My liver enzymes eventually normalized, and I was back to a two-drug treatment plan of ten milligrams of prednisone and 150 milligrams of Imuran daily. I was even able to discontinue taking cholestyramine, as the itching subsided when my liver enzymes returned to normal values.

It was a little strange having my fellow mother-baby nurses care for Kyle and me. They saw me in a whole new light. On one hand, I trusted them and knew I was being well taken care of. On the other hand, I didn't like my co-workers assessing the most intimate details of my postpartum recovery. I had had a fourth-degree episiotomy during Kyle's delivery, and sitz baths and Tylenol with codeine were the only things that got me through my postpartum pain. I closely watched how much Tylenol I took, since acetaminophen is hard on the liver. With liver disease, I am limited to two grams of acetaminophen a day (people with healthy livers can have up to four grams a day).

It was a big adjustment becoming parents. All new parents have one thing in common—we are a bunch of sleep-deprived zombies. Kyle kept us up all night. He appeared to be nocturnal; we weren't quite prepared for that. He also snored. *What kind of baby snores?* To quiet his snoring, we propped him up to sleep in his bouncy chair and moved the chair into the living room. I love sleep. I live for my afternoon naps and full-night sleeps. This bizarre schedule of waking every two to three hours was insane. Why do babies try to kill off their parents? Is it some kind of initiation into parenthood—only the strongest sleep-deprived parents will survive? Kyle seemed to have a ravenous appetite, thanks to the Edwards' family genes, and ate often, especially in the night. I broke one of the "rules" in the *What to Expect When You're Expecting* book: I fed Kyle rice Pablum at two months old just to keep his tummy full through the night. The trick worked superbly without any ill effects, and we got more than an hour or two of sleep each night.

In Canada, mothers get a year of maternity leave, if they choose to take it. Even fathers can take paternity leave. In the United States, mothers get only three months' maternity leave. Kevin and I both worked full-time, so I looked into sending three-month-old Kyle to daycare. During my first daycare "interview," I saw a baby in an automatic baby swing, alone in the corner of a room. Tears were running down his little cheeks, and no one was going over to console him. I made up my mind right then and there not to send my little boy to daycare. I went down to working only two twelve-hour night shifts a week. On the days when I had worked the night before, I would sleep stretched out on our comfy green couch, with Kyle sound asleep upon my chest. They were some wonderful snuggle times.

Our first year as parents went by in a blur. Kyle brought a lot of joy into our lives, and we had fun being his parents *most* of the time. Kevin and I had discussed moving back across the border, and so began Kevin's job search. He landed a job at the University of Waterloo as a software developer for the Herschel Space Telescope. Perfect, we thought. We would be able to move to Ontario. Only the job wasn't in Waterloo—it was in Groningen, Netherlands. I had always wanted to be a foreign exchange student in high school, and now I could fulfill my dream of living in Europe. Kevin gladly accepted the position, and we began googling Groningen. *Where was this city, anyway?*

Chapter 5

WONEN IN NEDERLAND

On January 2, 2006, we moved to the Netherlands, a country known for wooden shoes, tulips, windmills, cheese, and canals. Once we arrived at Schiphol Airport in Amsterdam, we took the train to Groningen—a two-hour and twenty-minute train trip. Our trip from Edmonton, where we'd spent Christmas with Kevin's family, to our new house in Groningen took us twenty-six hours and across eight time zones. Needless to say, we were exhausted and cranky and looking forward to sleeping in a bed.

One of Kevin's co-workers, Peter, met us at the train station and drove us to our new house. We arrived in the evening, so it was dark and we had no clue where we were. Peter showed us around our new house and helped bring in half of our luggage (because the other half of our luggage was lost in Frankfurt). It was a furnished three-storey row house and more modern than we had imagined.

The first thing we noticed with the house was the steep and narrow stairs. The stairs would never pass code in Canada. They were more like ladders with a meagre depth that accommodated less than half of my foot. We had to climb the stairs in the same way we would climb a ladder, clinging precariously to the upper steps with our hands or grabbing hold of the wall railing.

The second thing we noticed was our landlords' decorating tastes. It looked like they shopped at Ikea for their furniture. The couches and tables were very box-like and had that self-assembled look. There were hand-painted traditional African masks and tribal paintings on the walls. This house needed some redecorating . . . the scary masks had to go. The Dutch also have an obsession with houseplants, as we saw in our own house and neighbours' houses. Even the attic had cacti growing among the bookshelves and moving boxes.

We arrived with only a few suitcases containing essential items like clothes and toiletries. The rest of our belongings for the move were shipped from Lansing and were expected to arrive in mid-February. Until then, we had to survive with the few things we had packed on the airplane. Most of Kyle's toys were in moving boxes somewhere between the United States and the Netherlands. With all the potted plants scattered around the house, there was ample dirt for Kyle to dig in . . . and make a mess in, and eat.

We moved most of the plants to our garden in the backyard. As we learned, the Dutch covet their backyard gardens. Some neighbours kept beautifully manicured gardens with tulips and daffodils in perfect patterns. In our backyard, we had a wild rainforest of a magnolia tree, a plum tree, bamboo, herbs, and ferns lining a bricked path that stretched from one end of the backyard to the other. Weathered wooden patio furniture and terracotta pots could be seen among all the plants. There was even a wild hedgehog that lived underneath the ferns that we named Mr. Prickles.

We didn't own a car; we took the less expensive way to get around and biked everywhere. We biked in the rain, wind, and snow—we dressed for the occasion and away we went. Our house came with two rickety bikes with high handlebars, fenders, and three gears (which didn't work half the time). It was questionable how road-worthy Kevin's bike was. The Netherlands has the highest density of bikes in the world—a fact I had read in a Dutch newspaper. If you think it is difficult to find your car in the Walmart parking lot,

I urge you to try to find your bike among the thousands of bikes in the underground parking structures. People went to all sorts of trouble to distinguish their bike from others. I spray-painted my bike hunter green, painted white polka dots along the frame, and added star stickers to the fenders. Since we had little Kyle, we purchased a child's seat with a windshield for the front of my bike.

Cycling was a generally safe mode of transportation. The Netherlands is equipped with a network of cycling trails and bike lanes separate from the traffic. There are special traffic lights for cyclists at intersections, so cyclists don't have to cross the intersections with the cars. The only problem with this bike light system is that all cyclists in every direction cross at the same time when the light turns green. It is bicycle mayhem, and you have to carefully watch other cyclists so you don't wind up in an accident. I saw more people hit this way, and even witnessed two cyclists collide and spill all their groceries onto the middle of the intersection. I will admit that I too was involved in a few collisions, including a collision with a duck!

Our first challenge was learning to speak Dutch. We knew we were going to be living in the Netherlands for a few years, so we enrolled in a "Beginner's Dutch" course at Alpha College. It was easier to learn in class from a native speaker than from using Google Translate or listening to our *Beginner's Dutch* CD. I worked hard to learn the language. It wasn't so easy to pronounce the hard *G* sounds or roll the *R*s. I learned the basics, though, like how to ask where the bathroom was and how to ask for directions (which was important since I tend to get lost easily). I found the Dutch appreciated the fact I *tried* to speak their language, but I don't think they appreciated that I mutilated it. As much as I would try to converse in my broken Dutch, often people just spoke back to me in English. As soon as I knew they were willing and able to converse in English, I did likewise.

I joined a playgroup (speelgroep) in our neighbourhood and intently listened in on conversations between moms and their children, and sometimes attempted to engage in conversations with them. The playgroup always closed with all the moms sitting in a circle with their children and singing songs and eating biscuits. I hate to admit it, but the simple children's songs taught me many Dutch words.

The next challenge was to find a hepatologist who spoke English. Like in Canada and the United States, I had to find a family doctor (huisarts) first, and then have the huisarts refer me to a specialist. I was referred to hepatologist Dr. A.P. van den Berg at the Universitair Medisch Centrum Groningen (UMCG). UMCG is unlike any hospital I have ever been in. I wouldn't even call UMCG a hospital—it is a city within a city. The main lobby has palm trees, artwork, a small grocery store, a hair salon, a travel agent, and a beautiful water fountain. The glass ceilings are massively high and open in the summer. Each floor has a balcony patients can sit on for fresh air and a change in scenery. There was always an event happening in the lobby. One time, there was a children's fundraiser near the pediatric unit. I took Kyle to eat candy floss with the clowns and drive a little pedal car around the lobby. The hospital was so massive that the hallways were given street names. The liver clinic's address in the hospital was Fountain Street (Fonteinstraat) 17.

Dr. van den Berg was a wonderful hepatologist. I know I scared him over the years with some of my liver flare-ups and complications. I always liked that I could page him in an emergency, and he would respond to my call and set me up for hospital admittance. He took the time to explain things and his English was perfect. It turned out that most medical doctors spoke proficient English and there was no need for me to worry about important medical information being lost in translation.

My autoimmune hepatitis was quiescent during 2006. I had my blood tested every month and two routine abdominal ultrasounds each year to screen for liver cancer or other abnormalities. Dr. van den Berg also scheduled an outpatient gastroscopy for the fall of 2006, to check for esophageal varices—enlarged veins in the esophagus, and a complication of liver disease I had already experienced. I had several cherry-red spots (grade-two-to-three varices) in my stomach and esophagus. They were banded, meaning rubber rings were placed around the enlarged blood vessels to cut off circulation so they wouldn't bleed. This was a minor outpatient procedure, which I slept through with the help of sedation and pain medications.

Toward the end of 2006, Kevin and I discussed having another child. My pregnancy had gone so well with Kyle, and Kyle turned out just fine (as far as we could tell), so we decided to take the plunge. I knew from the get-go this time that I was pregnant because I was tracking my cycle. I didn't want to miss the first trimester again. The beginning of my pregnancy was uneventful. Then in February 2007, all hell broke loose—my liver was not happy with the new life growing inside me.

One afternoon, Kyle and I were visiting my friend Kelly and her son Julius. Kelly and I had formed a close friendship because she is American and Julius is the same age as Kyle. During the visit, I didn't feel so well, so Kelly watched Kyle while I slept in her spare room. I woke after a short nap and ran to the toilet and vomited a large amount of blood. This was the first time in my life I had vomited blood. I freaked out—vomiting blood is never a good thing. But I knew that meant my esophageal varices had ruptured. Thankfully, Kelly lived near UMCG, and I biked five minutes down the road to the emergency room, all the while vomiting blood into the plastic bag I had in hand. This automatically qualified me for my first hospitalization abroad.

I was assigned to a private room in the gastroenterology ward. I had an emergency gastroscopy that evening, and the doctor banded my five bleeding esophageal varices. With all the extra blood volume during pregnancy, I had developed portal hypertension. Portal hypertension is an increase in the pressure within the portal vein, which is the vein that carries blood from the digestive organs to the liver. The increase in pressure is caused by an increase in blood volume or by a blockage in the blood flow through the liver. Increased pressure in the portal vein causes varices (enlarged veins) to develop across the esophagus and stomach, to get around the blockage. The varices become fragile and can bleed easily, as in my case.

The banding stopped the bleeding, but I continued to vomit bile and dry-heave the entire night. At one point I placed my pillow on the bathroom floor and draped a blanket over myself, and slept next to the toilet. I had already left a trail on my way from my bed to the bathroom, and I didn't want my nurse to have to clean up after me again. Plus, my roommate snored and was keeping me awake. I yelled "niet snurken!" at her many times, but she continued to snore away. Maybe I was mispronouncing the words, or maybe she was a really sound sleeper. She certainly didn't wake. If I wasn't so nice, I would have bopped her with my pillow or given her a little nudge so she would roll over and quit snurken.

My first hospitalization was three days long. My throat was so sore from the gastroscopy and continual retching. I was exhausted from vomiting for nearly twenty-four hours and from lack of sleep. I wanted to go home to my own bed in the worst way. Kevin biked with Kyle to the hospital to escort me home. This is what I find funny: I biked home after this hospitalization, and after subsequent hospitalizations. Since we didn't have a car and the bus often made me nauseous, I preferred to bike. I liked being out in the fresh air; it settled my stomach and cleared my head from the hospital smell and stuffiness. I also had plenty of places to pull off the bike trail and be sick.

The variceal bleed was only the beginning of my pregnancy complications. I also experienced rectal bleeding because I had developed external and internal hemorrhoids. *Those are itchy and painful little buggers.* The worst part was that I didn't have any warning when the hemorrhoids were going to bleed. Thankfully, the first time occurred at home, but while dealing with it, I also had to calm Kyle down because seeing a trail of blood on the floor had frightened him. Plus, he had stepped in some of my blood and it was on his socks. He was crying and repeating in his sweet toddler voice, "Mommy hurt, oh, poor mommy." I tried to reassure him I would be okay, even though I didn't believe that myself. When I paged Dr. van den Berg and explained the situation, he scheduled me for an outpatient sigmoidoscopy the next day.

The endoscopy department knew me as "the pregnant woman with liver disease from Canada." They nicknamed me "Mevrow Canada." I was now four months along and very concerned with the effects of sedation on the baby. The doctor only gave me a minimal amount of Versed and Demerol, enough to relax me and provide a little pain control. Because I was not fully out, after the tube was inserted into my rectum, I could see the five large varices on the computer screen displayed above the gurney. The doctor placed a rubber band around each varice to strangle it to death.

Rectal bleeding became a nuisance. The further along I got in my pregnancy, the more frequent the bleeding episodes. I decided to join a prenatal fitness class at the Kardinge pool. After the first class, I exited the pool, and upon seeing blood on the pool deck, the instructor thought I was having a miscarriage and had me lie down in a medical room. She wanted to call the ambulance. I explained why it wasn't an emergency, but she didn't understand what I was saying in English, so I reverted to Dutch. *What is the word for haemorrhoids . . . oh yeah,* aambeien, *like on the hemorrhoid cream tube.* I told the instructor, "Ik ben oke, alleen bloed. Ik heb aambeien." *I am okay, only blood, I have hemorrhoids.*

I underwent repeated sigmoidoscopy procedures during my pregnancy, but I hated subjecting my baby to all the sedation and narcotics, so I drew the line after five scopes. This pregnancy was in no way like my first. I would have given up eating sweets and dealt with gestational diabetes again over these complications.

I was under the care of high-risk obstetrician Dr. Zeeman. She and I instantly bonded because she used to live in Texas and loved to converse in English. I felt genuinely comfortable with her because we didn't have any language barrier between us and she had a wonderful bedside manner.

Dr. Zeeman closely followed my pregnancy. I had an ultrasound every two weeks to assess for ascites (fluid in my abdomen), during which Dr. Zeeman also gave me a quick glance at my growing baby. It always gave me great pleasure to watch the baby's heart beat. At twenty weeks, Kevin and Kyle joined me for the gender-revealing ultrasound. When I saw the ultrasound, I beat Dr. Zeeman to the punch and said, "Yep, it's a girl." We couldn't have been more excited. In my mind I could see a little girl twirling around in a pink dress with her hair tied up in ribbons and bows. As I watched my baby on the ultrasound, I kept thinking, *A little girl to go shopping with, a little girl to have tea parties with.* Then I brought my mind out of the clouds and thought, *Please, God, let my daughter and me make it through this pregnancy.*

On July 19, Kevin's birthday, I felt absolutely rotten. The ascites was worsening and I was having trouble breathing. I was up to 182 pounds (I'd started at 132 pounds pre-pregnancy). I had only gained twenty-two pounds with Kyle, and now I had gained fifty pounds with my daughter and still had a month to go before my due date. I was in the midst of making Kevin a chocolate cake when I felt my body fading and giving up. After the cake was iced (yes, I managed to finish the cake), I slept the rest of the afternoon in my bed with Kyle snuggled up against my back. We managed to order pizza and celebrate Kevin's thirty-third birthday, but I went back to bed after he blew out his candles.

The next day, Friday, July 20, five weeks before my due date, Kevin went to work as usual, so it was just Kyle and me at home. Kyle was only two and a half years old and still napped, so I put him in his crib while I curled up in my bed. When I woke and sat up on the edge of the bed, I felt like I was going to die. I was woozy, weak, chilled, and burning up. I tried to crawl to the phone in my room, but I was too weak and shaky, so I lay on the hard, wood floor for a few minutes. When I finally crawled around the bed to the phone, I called a taxi and said it was an emergency and I had to get to the hospital. Then I called the *Verpleegafdeling verloskunde en gynaecologie* (obstetrics and gynecology ward) and asked to speak to Dr. Zeeman. She was on holidays. I couldn't think, my mind was foggy, so I told the secretary my name and said, "I am coming now." Whether the secretary understood me, I don't know, but I knew I had to get to UMCG immediately; something was wrong, I could feel it. I called Kevin and warned him I was on my way to the hospital. I told him to come get Kyle before coming to see me. *Kyle, oh dear, what was I going to do with my sleeping boy?* It took all the strength I had to get myself out the door to the taxi. There was no way I had the time or energy to pick up Kyle and wrestle him to the taxi. I left Kyle sleeping in his crib, locked the door, and asked the neighbour to keep an eye on him.

Taxis in the Netherlands aren't what you would expect. They are plush BMWs and the driver wears a suit and tie. Taxi drivers are highly skilled in manoeuvring through narrow cobblestone streets, herds of cyclists, and crowds of pedestrians. They have special hospital privileges and can park near the emergency room entrance, next to the ambulance parking space. We learned the hard way that it is always better to call a taxi than an ambulance to get to the emergency room in Europe. I was playing hockey and endured a concussion when I was hit hard by a tall, male Dutch player during a practice. I was taken to UMCG by ambulance. The ambulance cost 900 euros, whereas a taxi would have cost fifteen euros for the same distance travelled.

The taxi driver was very concerned with my condition and kept telling me he was driving fast and we were almost there. He even found a wheelchair and personally escorted me to the obstetrics and gynecology ward. I tipped him well. A midwife came and performed an ultrasound. The baby's heart rate was too fast, and my maternal fever was the cause. If I'd been in the United States or Canada, I'm sure the situation would have rendered an emergency C-section. In the Netherlands, births are usually au naturel. In fact, many women deliver at home with a midwife. My midwife was frightened by my autoimmune hepatitis, so she called in an obstetrician and an anesthesiologist to assess me for a C-section. Both doctors concurred that I was not a good candidate for a C-section because I had too much ascites, and this accumulation of abdominal fluid could endanger the baby if my abdomen was cut open. I also had another complication. The anesthesiologist figured with my abnormal, inadequate blood clotting that I was at risk of bleeding complications if he inserted an epidural into my spine. He didn't seem comfortable taking on my case. I was not at all in favour of having a C-section, and in no way did I want an epidural. I had delivered once au naturel, and I was prepared to do it again.

The midwife and I knew the baby needed to be delivered *now*. My baby was experiencing fetal distress, and I was very sick and had even started vomiting at this point. The nurse gave me paracetamol, but that only brought my forty degree Celsius fever down to 39.5. The midwife started me on IV Pitocin to induce labour. She also rubbed cervical ripening gel inside me to help thin my cervix in an effort to further induce labour.

After a rough night of dealing with a high fever, vomiting, and constant worry for the well-being of my daughter, I was dilated eight centimeters by late morning and almost ready to push. The labour and delivery team set me up for delivery in a large room equipped with everything from an incubator to a code cart. Kevin stayed near the head of my bed, stroking my hair and keeping me calm. It didn't take long for the urge to push to flash over me. The midwife didn't want me to push, however, because she didn't think I was having contractions. I was filled with too much ascites fluid for the contractions to register on the monitor. There was a lot of Dutch chit-chat going on, so I'm not sure about the whole story behind the midwife and nurses not believing I was ready to push. They left the room, so Kevin and I were alone when I shouted at him, "I need to push! Get the midwife." He told me to hold on and yelled down the hall for help. I needed to push and the baby was coming out. I think I told Kevin he was going to have to catch our daughter. It's lucky the midwife and nurses came running into our room when they did. They caught the baby with their bare hands.

Our little meisje (girl), Sarah Christine Edwards, was born on July 21, 2007, at 3:15 p.m. She was a little peanut, only 16.5 inches long and weighing five pounds three ounces. Sarah was so tiny because she was born slightly premature at thirty-five weeks. She was on the borderline of being able to stay with me or having to go to the neonatal intensive care unit—she managed to breathe on her own, but was underweight and small. We could keep her with us as long as she remained stable. Little Sarah was bald and blue-eyed with noticeably long fingers—Kevin's fingers. In the Netherlands it is customary at the birth of a baby to give the new parents a treat called *beschuit met muisjes*, which is a crispy, dry biscuit spread with butter and sprinkled with pink and white licorice-flavoured sprinkles (muisjes, or "little mice"). If I'd had a boy, the sprinkles would have been blue and white. I was too ill to eat, so Kevin enjoyed the treat.

I don't know what went wrong, but within an hour after delivery, I had to hand Sarah over to Kevin because I felt incredibly sick and had a sudden, violent bout of diarrhea and vomiting. This sudden loss of fluids made me light-headed, and I somehow slid onto the bathroom floor. I managed to reach for the red emergency cord. My nurse came in, saw me, and freaked out. She said a bunch of Dutch words and ran to get some help. A couple of nurses picked me up off the bathroom floor, undressed me, and showered me off. I was assisted back to the table and shook uncontrollably. I was cold so the nurses bundled me in warm blankets. They took my vitals and my temperature was forty-one degrees Celsius. The next thing I remember, a hepatologist (one of Dr. van den Berg's colleagues) was beside me, telling me he needed to obtain a sample of my ascites fluid because he suspected I had an infection. Thankfully I was pretty out of it when he stuck a needle into my lower abdomen. Within an hour, the doctor returned and said I had developed spontaneous bacterial peritonitis, which is a bacterial infection in the ascites fluid, and I was started on the IV antibiotic ceftriaxone.

I only remember bits and pieces of my stay in the postpartum room. I was pretty sick and in and out of consciousness. Sarah was in her bassinet next to my bed, where I could watch her angelic face. When she began to fuss, I tried to pick her up out of her bassinet and place her on my breast for feeding. The nurse came into my room and scolded me for not calling for help. Apparently, the nurse thought the antibiotics could enter my breast milk. But I knew from being a mother-baby nurse that ceftriaxone was safe to administer to breastfeeding mothers. I had a difficult time explaining that in Dutch to my nurse, so I just went along with my nurse's suggestion and gave Sarah a bottle. I was too sick to argue and too sick to care how Sarah was fed. I was just happy that she wasn't fussing anymore and had a full tummy.

Late that evening, the neonatologist made rounds and did a physical assessment on Sarah. Sarah had a heart murmur and needed an echocardiogram. While the neonatologist took Sarah for her echo, I had a chance to freshen up in the bathroom. While sitting on the toilet, I felt a very strange sensation. Sure enough, my uterus had prolapsed, and was now a large, pink balloon hanging outside my body. Understandably, I totally freaked. I pulled the red emergency cord. A male nurse rushed in. I didn't care that the nurse was male; I needed help. I don't think he had ever witnessed a real live prolapsed uterus—they aren't very common. He ran away. *Wait, where are you going . . . don't leave me here . . . I can't walk.* He returned with a female nurse, who explained to me that yes, it was a prolapsed uterus. *I know that, I've seen a prolapsed uterus in my patients . . . now please help me.*

The nurse assisted me back to bed. She elevated the lower portion of the bed and placed pillows on my hips to use gravity to assist in placing my uterus back inside, but that didn't really work and required the help of Dr. Zeeman, who apologized for missing Sarah's unexpectedly early birth. She told me to remain on bed rest for two days and keep my hips and legs elevated. *How was I going to get up and pee*, I wondered. *I bet someone is going to come catheterize me . . . not another medical procedure.*

I have inserted urinary catheters on many patients. It was one of the first skills I learned in nursing school. Now it was my turn to have a long plastic tube stuck in me. Even worse was the fact I had an audience of about ten medical students. Dr. Zeeman asked if the procedure (which wasn't as painful as I had imagined because Dr. Zeeman was an expert in catheterization) could be a teaching moment for her medical students because none of them had seen a prolapsed uterus, other than a textbook diagram. I only agreed because I was a perfect model for teaching students about a prolapsed uterus. I told the students, "Just so you know, babies ruin our bodies."

The only thing that got me through this whole ordeal was wanting to go home with my daughter and see Kyle again. *Oh sh**, where was Kyle??* I later discovered that, as I'd requested, Kevin had rescued Kyle from his crib shortly after I'd called him to say I was on my way to the hospital. Kyle was only alone for maybe thirty minutes and had remained sleeping the whole time.

Things got worse over the next couple of days. I swelled up and looked more pregnant than I had when I was actually pregnant. My liver enzymes were elevated, and each day more and more ascites filled my abdomen. A hepatologist was called in to deal with me. Apparently Dr. van den Berg missed all the excitement because he was on summer holidays. I was instantly started on IV Solu-Medrol to help control my liver flare-up. The hepatologist told me she needed to perform a paracentesis (abdominal tap). If I could have got up off the bed and locked myself in the bathroom, I would have. A paracentesis involves sticking a large needle into the abdomen and draining the ascites fluid. *Another freakin' needle, and a big one at that.* This was my first tap and I needed some hand-holding, so I called Kevin at home to come support me through this.

The hepatologist removed three litres of fluid (three kilograms or 6.6 pounds) from my abdomen. How disgusting! I instantly felt like I had delivered another baby. My abdomen was no longer huge and bloated. Not all the fluid was removed because the hepatologist was concerned that removing too much fluid too fast could send my body into shock. An IV Lasix infusion helped me excrete the rest of the fluid. I lost over forty pounds from the time of admission until the time of discharge—including, of course, weight loss from delivering Sarah. I was warned that the Lasix infusion was going to prevent me from breastfeeding Sarah because Lasix enters breast milk. If Sarah were to drink my milk, she too would receive a dose of Lasix and pee more, and we didn't need any more wet nappies to change.

Losing the fluid also helped treat my uterus problem. The ascites had put an extreme amount of pressure on my abdomen and worsened the prolapsed uterus. The urinary catheter was removed and I was allowed to move around again, which was good because I am not good at sitting still.

The whole time I was dealing with my problems, something more concerning, more important to me, was overshadowing my postpartum complications: Sarah wasn't with me. Dr. Zeeman requested, against my wishes, for Sarah to be transferred to the Verpleegafdeling Neonatologie—the neonatal intensive care unit (NICU). I couldn't effectively take care of Sarah in my state. I was in and out of consciousness and had to be on bed rest with my bottom elevated. Dr. Zeeman was also concerned with Sarah's weight and heart murmur. Sarah was underweight, five weeks premature, and not eating well. I knew wholeheartedly she needed to be in the NICU, but I desperately wanted her with me. She was my daughter, and I was supposed to take care of her. At least Kevin was able to give Sarah her first bath. But I was so out of it, I don't even remember it.

I suffered from postpartum depression in the hospital during my two-week stay. I felt like my heart was ripped out of my chest when Sarah was taken from me. I cried many tears. I was suffering from the physical complications from her birth, and seeing her and holding her helped me forget about my problems, reassured me that my physical suffering was worth it.

I was transferred from the obstetrics and gynecology ward to the gastroenterology ward on the third floor. I was constantly nagging the nurses to let me go see Sarah. I couldn't walk there myself because my uterus might fall out. My nurse finally agreed to wheel me to see Sarah. I sat in my wheelchair with my daughter in my arms for a couple of hours. I was able to feed her a bottle and change her nappy and clothes. All the pretty pink, frilly clothes my mom had shipped to us didn't fit Sarah. She was the size of a doll. My friend Kelly bought Sarah a preemie outfit, so I dressed Sarah in the onesie. Even that was a little large, but it was a whole lot cuter than the hospital gown.

Kevin arranged for Mom to fly from Toronto to the Netherlands. We desperately needed her help, and I wanted my mom. There's something comforting about having your mom around when you are sick. Kevin had neighbours and friends take Kyle for an hour or two when he came to visit Sarah and me at the hospital. But he needed full-time care for Kyle. Plus, I was going to need help once I was discharged. With Mom's arrival, things at home were more manageable for Kevin, and he was able to visit Sarah and me more often.

The day of discharge was much anticipated. There's no place like home. The hospital can be my place of work, fine, but I really hate being a patient there. Two weeks was a long time to be stuck indoors during the summer. The NICU was no longer the place for Sarah, since she was a healthy baby. Her heart murmur was no longer apparent or a concern; it was likely an innocent murmur that went away on its own. She had actually gained a few ounces by the time we were discharged. Her nurses told me she developed quite an appetite for Simulac formula. I may not have been able to breastfeed her because of the Lasix, but that didn't bother me. I was happy she was eating and gaining weight. However, I knew we had a long way to go before I could tie her hair up in ribbons and bows—she was completely bald.

My mom lived with us for six weeks. I was still recovering from my whole ordeal, and we couldn't have survived without her. Mom got up in the middle of the night and tended to Sarah's frequent feedings and dirty nappies. Because Sarah was so tiny, she had difficulty regulating her body temperature. We kept a warm water bottle against her back when she slept, like the nurses had done in the NICU. Sarah also needed to sleep with her wicker bassinet at a forty-five-degree angle with her head elevated because it helped keep formula in her stomach—she had a tendency to regurgitate her feedings.

In the Netherlands, we have the "baby police," otherwise known as the *consultatiebureau* (children's health clinic). Parents must visit a doctor and nurse to keep track of their child's growth and development from birth until age four. I always loved how the doctor and nurse would tell me my kids were too short. I had to laugh at that. Did they expect me to stretch them? The Dutch breed tall children, and my kids came from Canadian genes. I had no control over their height. Our family doctor, Dr. Wessling, also paid me a visit postpartum. This I liked—the family doctor, with her little black doctor's bag, visiting the patient at home. *Just like the olden days.* Dr. Wessling requested to see Sarah's room and thoroughly checked over our house. In a way I felt like she was spying on us, but she was only checking to see if our house was clean and safe for the children.

Dr. Wessling performed a postpartum physical exam on me. I lay on my bed as she checked my prolapsed uterus. I was still having problems with the "balloon" coming out. She told me she would refer me for pelvic floor therapy and recommended I have a pessary inserted (a plastic ring that fits inside the pelvic floor to hold the uterus in place). I found pelvic floor therapy sessions uncomfortable, so I attended only a few, but I did eventually have a gynecologist fit me for a pessary.

As much as I liked living in Europe, I did become quite home-sick. The rainy, dreary, grey skies certainly were depressing. I felt cooped up inside our damp house. It didn't feel like home because most of our belongings were in a storage unit in Belleville. The house was decorated to suit the landlords' taste, not ours (I did replace the African masks with the kids' artwork).

What helped with homesickness was making friends. We didn't just stick to making friends with other English-speaking expats. We made friends with our Dutch neighbours. Their kids and ours ran around the streets and played together until the streetlights came on, like we did as kids. Our large bay window in the kitchen overlooked the playground, so I would occasionally check that all the kids were safe and getting along. There were often older children to keep an eye on the younger children. It was a safe neighbourhood and we all looked out for our fellow neighbour.

The kids and I travelled back to Canada to visit family at least once a year, usually during summer holidays. Just a word of advice: Don't give kids Gravol. It doesn't make them sleepy, it makes them hyper monsters—I'm just saying.

Flights between Toronto and Amsterdam didn't come cheap, so I found a way to alleviate the costs. I was hired as an RN at the Belmont Long Term Care Facility in Belleville during the summer. It was a perfect arrangement. I was able to help cover summer vacations and sick time while keeping my nursing skills fresh. I loved the staff and residents. It was a good job and fit well with my schedule—not to mention that I missed the working world! I had a difficult time being a stay-at-home mom with the kids. I had worked as a nurse in the United States, and now I was home changing nappies, cleaning up after the kids, and wiping snot from their noses. I was surrounded by their constant noise and messes, and it really drove me crazy sometimes.

My medical complications did not end after Sarah's birth. My liver enzymes were never normal, but they were fairly stable while I was on ten milligrams of prednisone and one hundred milligrams of Imuran. Dr. van den Berg also added ten milligrams of the beta-blocker propranolol, three times a day, to my medication schedule to lower the pressure in my hepatic portal veins, thus reducing the likelihood I would endure additional rectal bleeds. However, in February 2011, I endured the worst rectal bleed yet. Kyle was at school, so only Sarah and I were home. We were getting ready for a jaunt to the market in the Centrum to purchase fruit and fish for supper. As I was putting on my jacket, I felt that familiar wet, warm trickle down my legs. *Not again . . . I don't have time for this.* I ran to the bathroom and stripped down in the bathtub. As I was undressing, I saw a few large blood clots the size of my fist slide down into the tub and felt faint. I sat down, half-naked, and yelled for Sarah to bring me the phone. I urgently paged Dr. van den Berg. I knew this was an emergency. I was losing a lot of blood and feeling like I wanted to go to sleep. I wasn't thinking straight and I didn't think of protecting three-year-old Sarah from seeing me covered in blood. But Sarah didn't seem frightened, only concerned. She asked, "Mommy, are you okay?" I told Sarah we were going to take a taxi to the hospital. Sarah went downstairs and dragged my shoes and coat up to the bathroom. That was really sweet of her to help me get ready, even if she dropped my coat in a pool of blood on the floor.

When we arrived by taxi at UMCG—my home away from home—ER staff admitted me right away because I was bleeding on the floor of the waiting room. Nothing gets the attention of ER staff faster than someone saying "I have chest pain" or someone who is bleeding profusely. I was admitted to the gastroenterology unit once again. This time I shared a wardroom with three other patients—two women and a man. *A man...is this even allowed?* Apparently in the Netherlands, the rooms are co-ed. At least he remembered to put the toilet seat down. One of my roommates was waiting for a liver transplant.

Here I was, back in the hospital for a one-week stint at the very expensive "hotel." I was given IV labetalol, another medication to lower the blood pressure in my hepatic veins and help treat the portal hypertension. I was also put through the sigmoidoscopy rig-marole, and my rectal varices were banded again. By this point my feeling toward having a scope had evolved from deathly fear to *let's get it over and done with, and me out of the hospital ASAP.*

I had racked up tens of thousands of euros in health care costs, and our health care coverage was insanely complicated. The University of Waterloo tried to cover our health expenses as if we were on a very long vacation. This basic health insurance did not cover pre-existing conditions such as my autoimmune hepatitis. To receive the extended medical coverage provided by the university, we would participate in a convoluted process involving rejection letters, phone calls, exchange rates, and mailed and re-mailed cheques. Each medical claim would take about a year to process from the time we got the bill to the time it was paid.

We also had problems with the medical billing practices. The Dutch have an electronic health records and insurance system for everyone, so mailing out bills for services was not their usual prac-tice. It wasn't uncommon for us to wait more than a year to receive a bill from a hospital or doctor's office. However, our Canadian insur-ance providers required that all claims be submitted within a year of service. You can't submit a claim without a bill . . .

We were constantly on the phone with UMCG or Dr. Wessling's office to reassure them that yes, they would get paid, but they had to wait for the insurance company to pay us first. I kept a spreadsheet and a cardboard box with copies of medical claims because this con-fusing process had a lot of glitches. We were still trying to get the insurance company to pay thousands of euros to UMCG even after we moved back to Canada.

At my last appointment with Dr. van den Berg before we returned to Canada, he wrote a referral letter to the Francis Family Liver Clinic at Toronto Western Hospital. In his letter he stated: "Apart from the episode of decompensation after the pregnancy, Mrs. Jowett's liver disease has been relatively stable. In view of her MELD scores in the range of thirteen to fourteen, we did not screen for transplantation as yet because under the MELD system, scores of twenty or above are required in the Netherlands to get a good donor offer, and transplantation. Her MELD range would probably not offer a survival benefit. Apart from this, Mrs. Jowett would not opt for a transplant at this stage. It is my feeling that the lady will not escape a transplant, however. 'Stable' as she may be, decompensation will easily occur when some complication (a variceal bleed, an episode of pneumonia) should come along. Personally, I would suggest initiating screening after she has settled in Canada again, and evaluate the possibility of having a deceased or living donor."

Chapter 6

VERHUIZEN—MOVING

In May 2011, we took on the challenge of moving from Groningen back to Canada. Moving down the street is stressful enough; moving across the Atlantic Ocean was a three-month-long migraine that wouldn't give up. It took three months to pack all the things we had accumulated over the last five and a half years. *Where did all this stuff come from?* We had arrived in Groningen with so few belongings, and now we had towers of boxes in our living room.

We packed everything ourselves, which made for a lot of work. We couldn't let the moving company pack because our belongings were interspersed with the landlords' belongings. I'm sure the landlords wouldn't have been too happy with us if we'd shipped their scary African masks back to Canada. It was sad, in a way, to see the boxes accumulate. They were a reminder that our living-abroad phase was over and there was no turning back now. At the same time, we were excited and ready to embark on a new adventure and move back home to Canada—back to the white, cold, snowy nation with Tim Hortons on every corner and being able to say "eh" without getting made fun of.

Our family flew from Amsterdam to Toronto in late May. My parents took the kids to Belleville while Kevin and I went on a house-hunting expedition in the Waterloo region of southern Ontario. We had three weeks to find a house before Kevin had to return to the Netherlands for work and to let the movers into our house there. Talk about stressful! After viewing over fifty houses (which all started to look alike after a while), we settled on a two-storey house in a quiet, family-friendly neighbourhood in Kitchener. We chose a house close enough for Kevin to bike to the University of Waterloo. We also chose a house that didn't need much in the way of renovations and had a sizable backyard that was perfect for a trampoline, vegetable garden, and flowerbeds. It was a bonus that the backyard was sloped—we could envision a toboggan hill for our kids.

We took possession of our house in July, and the kids and I were reunited with Kevin when he officially moved back to Canada in August. He came back in time to help with the move. We rented the largest U-Haul truck we could legally drive to move our possessions from the storage unit in Belleville to our house in Kitchener. The truck was filled to capacity and then some. Between everything we had in our storage unit and everything we accumulated in the Netherlands, we had double and even triple of some items. We immediately had a yard sale—that was one way to meet our new neighbours!

Luckily, my liver disease was quiet during this international transition, because there wasn't any time to visit the hospital, and I didn't have doctors in place and wasn't yet familiar with the Waterloo Region's hospitals. I didn't have provincial health care coverage (OHIP) yet because there is a three-month waiting period to obtain OHIP coverage after residency is established, but I still had private health care coverage through the University of Waterloo (I always made sure I had health care coverage after that burnt foot incident). When we applied for OHIP at a Service Ontario Centre, the representative pleasantly gave us the organ donation form to fill out. This was the first time I realized the old organ-donor paper cards were no longer valid. Without hesitancy, I checked the box to donate all organs and tissues. This was Kevin's first time registering his consent for organ and tissue donation.

In the fall, Kyle began grade two and Sarah started junior kindergarten. With the kids off to school, I began my job hunt. There was a part-time cardiology job posted at St. Mary's Hospital in Kitchener. I hadn't worked in cardiology since my time at Sparrow Hospital in Lansing. I dusted off my cardiology nursing textbooks and did a quick review before my interview. I could barely remember what a normal sinus EKG strip looked like.

I like cardiology because most cardiac patients are not going to get me sick with a communicable disease. Cardiac patients are often admitted because they are in heart failure, have endured a cardiac arrest, or require a pacemaker or defibrillator. They aren't usually carrying an infection that is going to invade my weak immune system. Cardiology also offers a lot of job security. Heart disease and stroke are two of the three leading causes of death in Canada. In fact, every seven minutes in Canada, someone dies from heart disease or stroke.

I have never had the desire to work in a gastroenterology unit or areas that involve working with people with liver disease. You would think I would have gravitated toward helping patients like myself because we share common ailments. On the contrary, I do not like seeing liver disease patients become ill and seeing what is likely going to happen to me in the future. When I was a nursing student, one of my first patients had liver disease. He died from alcoholic liver cirrhosis, and seeing him suffer from end-stage liver disease really hit home.

The interview went well and I landed the job. I unpacked my scrubs and stethoscope and waded back into the working world in October 2011. I felt like a new grad all over again—nervous, unsure, and intimidated. My first day in the inpatient cardiology unit, 3 East, was overwhelming. I didn't know where any of the supplies were; it was like a scavenger hunt. The syringes were in one closet in the bottom storage bin, and the needles for the syringes were in another closet fifty meters down the hall, on another cart.

The funny thing was, the nurses knew where all the supplies were kept. The sticky EKG buttons were in packages scattered here, there, and everywhere. I scored big if I found a package with five buttons, enough to put all the EKG leads on a patient. I also couldn't figure out the numbering system for the rooms. The room numbers went from 157-1 to 191-2 without any particular order. When I had a patient in room 157-1 and a patient in room 190-2, I had to hike (and sometimes run) kilometers a day from one end of our unit to the other. I managed to survive the first week of twelve-hour day shifts with countless bottles of Coca-Cola and a few of the chocolates and treats that always seem to be in the break room. I needed this sugar rush because I didn't have time for my afternoon nap. When one or two in the afternoon struck, I was used to crawling up under the covers for at least an hour's sleep.

There were many times I would come home and complain to my husband about how much I hated my job. I was annoyed with having to scavenge for supplies. I was annoyed with the fact we seldom got breaks during our twelve-hour shift—there was no time to eat or drink, and we weren't allowed food or drink at the nurses' station. I was annoyed with the amount of charting and that I did not have enough time for bedside care of patients. And I was absolutely overwhelmed when I had six patients to care for (plus my co-worker's five or six patients when she went on break) who were spread from one end of our unit to the other. The job was "too much" and I wasn't used to the pace. I was used to eating and peeing when I wanted and putting my feet up for a rest when I was tired. I wondered what I'd been thinking, wanting to go back to work. Being a stay-at-home mom wasn't so bad after all. Kevin was always prepared for me to come home in a grumpy mood and say, "That's it, I'm quitting."

I didn't quit. I wanted to hand in my notice, but I didn't. *I'm not a quitter*, I would tell myself. *What doesn't kill you makes you stronger, isn't that how the cliché goes?* Actually, what got me through those first few weeks on the job were my co-workers. If I didn't have such helpful, caring, and wonderful co-workers, I would have left. The job was daunting, but with the help of my co-workers, I survived twelve-hour shifts without losing my mind. They lent a hand when my patient load was too demanding. They helped me work through problems and answered questions when I struggled. We work as a close-knit team and have the utmost confidence in one another. We depend on that to ensure a good outcome with every patient and to help us get through each hectic shift—well, that, and the treats in the break room.

My co-workers also let me nap when I had a break, which was the other thing that got me through my twelve-hour shifts. Twelve hours is a long time to work, even for a healthy person. I napped on the picnic table benches in the grassy area next to the hospital. I napped on the arched bench near the donation plaques at the hospital entrance (when the smokers weren't there). When it was raining or cooler outside, I would nap on the couch in the team room or rest my head on the table in the break room. I can nap anywhere, anytime. When I was seventeen, I once fell asleep on a bench at Disney World while crowds of people walked by.

I worked part-time but signed up for additional weekend shifts, or shifts on days the kids were both in school. My part-time job was really full-time, but without the benefits. Like with any new job, the more experience I gained, the more confidence I developed, and the easier the job became.

When we moved to Ontario, we were told finding a family doctor is tricky. There is a shortage of doctors in many places in Ontario, and most doctor's offices are not accepting new patients. Waiting lists for new patients are long. One doctor's office near our house had a three-year wait. *No wonder so many patients use the ER as their family doctor.* I ended up finding a family doctor through work—one of the perks of working at a hospital. There was a bulletin posted at our nurses' station advertising that the Andrew Street Family Health Centre was opening a new practice of family doctors. I set up an appointment with Dr. Art Winter for a family visit. I knew Dr. Winter and I would establish a close relationship. Chronically ill patients tend to visit their doctors frequently. I didn't expect Dr. Winter to be a liver disease specialist, but I knew I would need to visit him for prescription renewals, blood tests, and any other problem that might arise. I also knew our family needed a doctor for vaccinations and minor ailments.

Dr. Winter was a new grad, which meant he was young, up to date on current medical issues, and likely going to stay in practice for a long time. He is knowledgeable, takes the time to listen, and isn't intimidating—all the qualities I look for in a doctor. We were blessed to find such a wonderful doctor. And I was relieved that the health centre's staff were able to squeeze us in for last-minute appointments. I'm a walking medical disaster at times, so this accommodation was a plus.

Having a family doctor is fine for most people, but I needed a team of specialists to keep my engine running. My liver wasn't getting any younger and I wasn't getting any better, so I went back to the Francis Family Liver Clinic at Toronto Western Hospital. After a couple of changes in hepatologists (Dr. Heathcote retired and the doctor I was passed on to moved), I was assigned to Dr. Hemant Shah. Dr. Shah is a clinic director at the Francis Family Liver Clinic and an assistant professor. His clinical focus is viral liver disease, and he maintains a busy teaching practice. I liked Dr. Shah right away, as he is a warm, well-spoken, and very knowledgeable doctor. He included me in discussions about my liver disease, explained what was going on, and answered my questions.

My liver disease was quiescent for the most part, so it was easy to manage my condition. I made my monthly blood donation to the lab to keep tabs on my liver enzymes. My liver enzymes were never normal, but they weren't significantly elevated either. I was on a stable dosing of ten milligrams of propranolol three times a day, ten milligrams of prednisone and one hundred milligrams of Imuran daily. I felt great. I worked my twelve-hour shifts several times a week. I played in a recreational women's hockey league. I biked five-kilometer to work and home each shift. I was a mom to Kyle and Sarah, who certainly kept me physically active. I played in the park, gardened, and ran around the backyard with the kids. Life to me was normal, just the way I liked it.

Chapter 7

NURSE OR PATIENT

As a registered nurse, I have rocked the sweetest newborn baby to sleep after he screamed for hours while withdrawing from his mother's heroin addiction. I have sat on the bed next to a mother who just delivered a stillborn baby and cried as she shared how excited she was to be delivering her first daughter and how things did not go as planned. I have joined a family in saying goodbye to their eighty-two-year-old father and husband with advanced heart failure. I get so much satisfaction from being able to make a positive impact on someone's life, even for a short period of time. Nursing is a fulfilling career with good pay and the added benefit of taking care of someone vulnerable and, in most cases, helping that person feel better and go home.

Nursing is definitely my true calling. I would never have guessed that I would enter a profession that involved needles, but my life has revolved around hospitals and doctors since I was thirteen-years-old. It was only fitting that I became part of the medical profession. I feel that I have learned things as a patient that have helped me become the nurse I am today. Knowing what it feels like to have a colonoscopy, and to prepare for it by drinking the solution that cleans out the bowels, allows me to empathize with my patients and makes it easier to answer procedure-specific questions. Having had many IV infusions, I am able to understand how difficult it is for patients to drag their IV pole while quickly trying to navigate their way to the toilet in an unfamiliar room.

In June 2012, life threw me a curveball, and I lost my grip. One morning I woke up and felt horrible, like I was plagued by the flu. I was cold yet had a fever of forty-one degrees Celsius. I was achy all over and had a pounding headache. My body felt like it was drained of life, and I lay on the couch cocooned in a fleece blanket. I knew it wasn't the flu, something didn't feel right. I couldn't put a finger on it, but it felt like something deep down inside wanted to give up. I had no energy, not even enough energy to eat or get dressed. *When I don't eat, that means I'm really sick.* Kevin took the kids to school and tucked me back into bed with my heated cherry-pit bag and a glass of water. He set the portable phone on my nightstand to call Dr. Winter when the office opened. Most people would take Tylenol, sleep off their illness, and head back to work in a day or two. When I get sick, I get sick for weeks. Tylenol doesn't always break my fever, and my liver enzymes often spike. Things can go badly quickly, so I don't let any illness slide.

Dr. Winter was not in the office that day, but the office was able to fit me in for an appointment right away with his colleague, Dr. Lubitz. I was still fevered at forty-one degrees Celsius, and that was after taking an extra-strength Tylenol a couple of hours before my appointment. I was flushed, restless, and achy. Some mild right upper abdominal pain also accompanied my symptoms. I just wanted Dr. Lubitz to magically make me better. *Isn't there a pill for that?* Since the source of my fever was unknown, Dr. Lubitz called the ER at Grand River Hospital in Kitchener and gave them the heads-up that I was on my way.

I was assessed by the triage nurse and advised to wear a yellow paper mask in case I was contagious. I knew I was in for a bit of a wait, but I hoped Dr. Lubitz's call to the ER would expedite the process. A lab technician with a fancy cart full of colour-coded blood vials and needles approached me. She brought me into a little corner room and took blood. The first order of business was figuring out the cause of my fever.

I went back to the crowded waiting room and tried not to watch the clock, but after four hours, I was getting impatient. I was uncomfortable and sick, but thanks to my ability to nap anywhere, anytime, I dozed off for about an hour with my head kinked forward, slouched in the chair. I'd expected a long wait, but not as long as this. *This* was ridiculous, so I left. Kevin and the kids picked me up and drove me home. I cocooned myself back into a blanket on the couch. It was more comfortable to rest there than in the ER. I debated what to do: return to the ER or stay home? I was feeling like rubbish and knew I needed medical attention, so I drove myself back to the ER shortly before midnight and checked back in. The kicker is, *my chart was still in the pile of charts for patients waiting to be seen. Staff didn't even know I was gone for over four hours.* I think I could have died in the waiting room and staff would not have noticed. The triage nurse checked my vitals again. I still had a 40.5 degree Celsius fever. She told me my chart was second from the top and the wait wouldn't be too much longer. I didn't believe her of course. I waited a total of ten hours and was never seen.

Around 2 a.m. I left and went home. I remember feeling discouraged and angry—what did it take for the ER staff to take me seriously and help me? I kept getting bumped by people entering the ER who were sicker than I was, or who had extensive injuries. I know there is a prioritization system in the ER; as a nurse I've floated to the ER many times. I was so desperate to be seen that I had considered faking chest pain during my wait.

Around suppertime the next day, I once again attempted to seek medical help. This time Kevin took me to the ER at St. Mary's Hospital. I was hoping that I could speed up the waiting process because I was an insider. When a nurse appeared through the sliding door and announced my name after "only" two hours, I pointed to myself and said, "You mean me?" Like there was another Christine Jowett in the waiting room. Maybe it did help that I was staff.

The ER nurse started an IV and began a normal saline infusion, the usual practice in the ER. I tried to weasel my way out of another blood draw because I had had blood drawn in the Grand River ER. It didn't work. St. Mary's Hospital needed their own set of labs. The results showed my platelets were low at thirty-nine (normal is 150 to 400) meaning I had thrombocytopenia. Big word, I know, but that was one of my diagnoses. With low platelets, I was prone to bleeding complications because platelets are needed to help clot blood. I also had a low white blood cell count at 1.6 (normal is 4.5 to 10.0). A low white blood cell count is called leukopenia. This meant I was at risk of developing an infection, and it also meant I couldn't fight whatever was afflicting me.

The ER doctor recommended I remain hospitalized until the source of my fever could be identified. And just like that, I became a patient on 3 East—the very place I worked. I waited in the ER until 2 a.m., when there was an empty bed available in a private isolation room. Our inpatient cardiology unit primarily houses cardiac patients, but we also accept medical patients when there are not any beds available on the medical floors. I'm glad it worked out this way. I not only got a private room, I was also taken care of by nursing friends I trusted. Because I was staff, my electronic chart was labelled *confidential*. I didn't want just anyone snooping into my medical records and learning personal things about me that could turn into hospital gossip. Most of my co-workers knew I had autoimmune hepatitis—that was no secret. I had to switch shifts with other nurses so I could make it to medical appointments. Besides sleeping during breaks, I was sometimes jaundiced and often retained fluid in my abdomen and legs—telltale signs of liver disease. It's difficult to hide medical symptoms from nurses, and before I had a chance to inform my co-workers of my disease, many of them had already figured me out.

The nurse assigned to me did a double take when she walked into my room and realized who her patient was. She jokingly asked, "Christine . . . is this your way of calling in sick?" My nurse didn't have to do much in the way of an admission assessment. She already knew about my medical history and most of my social history since we were friends. The admission assessment can take over an hour to complete when patients have a whole story to share, carry a pharmacy in their purse, or aren't able to answer questions accurately.

It's a funny thing when you're forced to see things in a different light. I wasn't the nurse anymore, I was the patient. What cracked me up was the reaction of patients when they saw me in pajamas pushing an IV pole down the hallways. Many did a double take and stopped to ask if I was okay. One elderly man asked with hesitancy, "Weren't you my nurse a couple of days ago?" Then he commented, "You must be here undercover, no nurse would want to be a patient."

I continued to endure fevers, chills, and abdominal pain. But the weird thing was, I was only fevered between 12:30 and 2 a.m., and 7 and 10 a.m. The rest of the day, I didn't have a fever and didn't feel too bad. *Why this trend?*

When I was fevered, my nurse friends would bring me ice cream and popsicles from the staff room freezer. They spoiled me with treats and I loved it! When I was given a meal tray that I didn't find appealing, staff would exchange it for a different one from the food cart. Some nurses brought in DVDs for me to watch on my computer. Others would bring me frozen lemonade or a muffin from the Tim Hortons downstairs. When I had trouble sleeping at night because of snoring patients and beeping pumps, I would sit at the nurses' station and visit. Sometimes my co-workers put me to work. I spent one evening stapling together patient handouts.

When I was first admitted, my liver enzymes were only slightly elevated. But after eight days with a fever, my liver enzymes became alarmingly elevated. Whatever was causing my fever was affecting my liver. Or vice versa—maybe this liver flare-up was causing the fever. My body was an unsolved mystery. Dr. Harry Wu immediately increased my prednisone dosage to fifty milligrams daily to combat my liver flare-up. He ordered a battery of tests to figure out what was going on. I had an abdominal ultrasound and abdominal CT, a colonoscopy and gastroscopy, and I even underwent a liver biopsy. My body was bruised and battered from all the poking and prodding, and Dr. Wu was no further ahead in trying to uncover the cause of my fever and illness.

Even so, I learned more about the inner workings of my body during my two-week hospitalization than I cared to know. Tests showed that my spleen was enlarged, I had two gallstones in my gallbladder, there was a blood clot in my splenic vein causing a partial occlusion, there was a small amount of ascites throughout my abdomen and pelvis, and I had low platelet and low white blood cell counts. The liver biopsy revealed active chronic hepatitis (activity-grade three out of four) and fibrosis (stage four out of four; definite cirrhosis or scarring). I knew my condition was worsening and it was just a matter of time before I would end up in end-stage liver disease. A liver transplant was inevitable. The question was, how much longer could I live with my own liver? Months? Years?

My fever remained undiagnosed. I was tested for many, many viral and bacterial infections, including CMV (Cytomegalovirus), EBV (Epstein-Barr virus), Lyme disease, meningitis, West Nile virus, and influenza. I didn't test positive for anything, so I was given a broad-spectrum antibiotic for one week in case I had an unidentified bacterial infection, or developed one, since I had a low white blood cell count.

The fifty milligrams of daily prednisone slightly lowered my liver enzymes, but they remained elevated. I was taken off Imuran because it can cause low numbers of white blood cells and platelets. I was given one unit of pooled platelets to help increase my platelet count, and two units of fresh frozen plasma to help my blood clot properly, but my counts never increased with these infusions.

Each day, I used my staff account to log in to Meditech, the hospital electronic charting system, to look up my daily labs and test results. I felt like I was spying on myself. I did sign a medical records release form so I wouldn't get in trouble for accessing my confidential medical records.

My fever broke the day before I was discharged, and after I finished my seven-day course of IV antibiotics, I was allowed to go home. My discharge summary stated that my diagnosis was *Fever NYD* (Not Yet Diagnosed). I likely had a liver flare-up, and my fever was a result of the flare-up, but that was just speculation by the doctors. After this hospitalization, my autoimmune hepatitis was more difficult to control despite higher doses of prednisone. Dr. Shah, my hepatologist, put me back on Imuran, which lowered my liver enzymes a little, although they still remained quite elevated.

Also, after I was discharged, my ascites worsened. My belly looked like that of a six-month-pregnant woman. I could see it grow each day and felt fluid sloshing around inside. Even my ankles and feet swelled. I was prescribed two diuretics to combat the fluid retention. I weighed myself daily to make sure the diuretics were working. Each kilogram lost meant I lost one litre of fluid. Since I'm a nurse, Dr. Shah allowed me to "play around" with my diuretic dosing based on my weight loss or gain. I was careful not to exceed a weight loss of greater than one kilogram per day.

I had biweekly blood tests while on diuretics to assess for electrolyte imbalances, renal insufficiency, and dehydration—some of the side effects of diuretics. I limited the amount of fluid I consumed to eight 250-millilitre cups of fluid per day. This was difficult to do with the summer heat. Now I knew why heart failure patients complained when we restricted their fluid intake. I also conformed to a sodium-restricted diet. I was allowed two grams of sodium per day. This wasn't easy to get used to. I had to read every food product label to familiarize myself with the sodium content. One cup of 2 percent milk has 130 milligrams of sodium, and two slices of white Wonder Bread have 300 milligrams of sodium. I was doomed; sodium is in everything. I was going to have to become a vegetarian and fruitarian—good thing we grow our own fruits and vegetables in our garden.

Over the next year, from July 2012 until June 2013, I battled with my liver disease. Scar tissue from cirrhosis had replaced healthy liver tissue, preventing my liver from functioning properly. The scar tissue blocked normal blood flow from my intestines through the liver. Without proper blood flow, the pressure increased in the portal vein system—the veins that supply the liver with blood—causing portal hypertension. The resulting ascites caused abdominal swelling to the extent that patients at work would often ask how far along I was, much to my dismay. My enlarged spleen caused my navel to protrude outward, adding to the pregnant look. The low platelet count meant my blood did not clot properly, and I bruised easily (I once had a doctor tell me I looked like a battered woman). My fluid-swollen legs and feet gave me chubby Fred Flintstone feet after I worked a twelve-hour shift. My eyes and skin were jaundiced; my husband said I had Marge Simpson's skin tone. My skin, particularly my chest, was covered in small red spots and tiny lines called spider angiomas (broken blood vessels). Multiple gallstones caused such intense pain to radiate from the right side of my abdomen to my right shoulder and into the middle of my back that I had to take morphine to deal with it. In the weeks prior to my transplant, I developed mild encephalopathy (altered brain function). I knew there were serious problems when I forgot to pick up Sarah from school on more than one occasion.

Dr. Shah kept a close eye on me. I saw him during office visits every three months, and we would chat over the phone when medication changes had to be made. I was patched up with higher dosages of medications, particularly prednisone.

My liver and I had a love-hate relationship. My liver wanted to throw in the towel and quit working. My body and mind wanted to fight to live, but with each illness I acquired, I felt my physical self become weaker and weaker. One simple cold would last a couple of days with Kevin and the kids, whereas my cold would linger for weeks and elevate my liver enzymes. I remember telling my family and friends that I predicted by the time I turned forty-years-old, I would need a liver transplant.

I'm not a quitter, and I wasn't about to let my liver disease be the cause of my death. I needed what little function my liver had left to keep me alive until I was sick enough to be evaluated for a transplant. Organs are made available to the sickest patients, and I wasn't quite there yet. While waiting to become sick enough to be listed for transplantation, I tried to enjoy life as best I could and not to act sick. I tried to live as normally as possible—if you call napping every day and sleeping ten to twelve hours a night normal.

I also often looked in the mirror at my unscathed abdomen. I knew in the very near future it would bear a lifelong scar. I took a picture of my abdomen and tucked the picture away to remind myself of what I once looked like.

Chapter 8

TRANSPLANT WORK-UP . . .
IS IT TIME FOR A NEW LIVER?

I had lived twenty-six years with my autoimmune hepatitis, so it was no shock to me when Dr. Shah referred me to a transplant surgeon and to the Pre-Transplant Liver Clinic at the University Health Network in Toronto. The liver I was born with was barely functioning, run down, and ready to be placed in a pickle jar labelled "surgical waste."

The organ transplant evaluation process began with meeting the transplant surgeon at the end of May 2013 to discuss the nitty-gritty surgical details. Sarah accompanied me to the appointment because she was in alternate-day kindergarten and it was her day off. We waited, and then waited some more. As we all know, doctors are *never* on time. It was difficult to keep Sarah occupied during the wait. I should have packed a colouring book and crayons. Instead, I kept her busy playing "I spy" with the limited colours in the tiny waiting room. Dr. Paul Grieg entered the room and gave me a welcoming handshake. He acknowledged Sarah with a smile and asked how old she was. She shyly told him she was five.

After examining me, Dr. Grieg helped me off the exam table because the ascites made it hard to push myself into a sitting position. We sat together at the little computer desk. He took a piece of blank paper from his desk drawer and a pen from his lab coat pocket, and drew a picture of a liver. He explained that a liver transplant is performed with a duct-to-duct approach (my bile duct attached to the donor bile duct), and how my liver would be removed and the donor liver transplanted.

He drew a picture of the incision, and then showed me on my abdomen with his index finger the approximate size and location of the incision. As Dr. Grieg moved his finger along my abdomen, he said, "The incision resembles either a peace sign or Mercedes Benz sign. How you see it depends on what stage of life you are in." This was the first time the incision had been described to me, and Dr. Grieg's demonstration confirmed what I already knew: it would be large and ugly.

Dr. Grieg also explained that I would no longer have my gallbladder after a liver transplant, as the surgeon would perform a cholecystectomy during the transplant surgery. That was good news; it would be a bonus that I would not have to experience those excruciatingly painful gallbladder attacks post-transplant.

We discussed the possible complications associated with surgery: bleeding, infection, rejection of my new liver, lack of function of my new liver. None of these possible complications scared me until he listed *death* as one of them. *I'm not going to die*, I thought. *I'm getting a new liver so I can live.*

Being the inquisitive patient I am, I wrote a list of questions before the appointment and jotted down the answers Dr. Grieg provided:

Will my spleen shrink after transplant?

It may shrink about 30 percent in size because you will no longer have portal hypertension (high blood pressure in the portal veins).

What will be done with the clot in the splenic vein?

If it isn't causing any complications, we will leave it.

Will my hernia be repaired?

You have a small umbilical hernia that may or may not be repaired during surgery. The transplant team will likely refer you for a hernia repair six or more months after transplant. If the hernia is causing you severe discomfort, then a surgeon may repair your hernia sooner. You may find that once you lose the ascites and your spleen regresses, the hernia no longer causes you discomfort. For now, wear a pregnancy belt or some type of abdominal support.

Will I be in a lot of pain post-op?

Your nurses will make sure your pain is controlled with narcotics. If you experience pain, make sure you tell your nurse. You will be given IV narcotics and likely a pain pump.

How long does it take to recover?

Every patient is different in terms of length of recovery. Generally we find patients feel better in three to six months.

I could have gone on all day asking questions, but I would have kept his other patients waiting (and I am sure they had been waiting long enough). I had enough answers to mentally prepare myself for the inevitable transplant.

My first visit to the Pre-Transplant Clinic at Toronto General Hospital was on Tuesday, June 25, 2013. While sitting with Sarah (again, it was a non-school day for her) in the crowded waiting room, I was scared and tense because there were so many unknowns. *Would I get sicker before I got better? Was I going to be accepted for transplant? How long would I have to wait for a new liver?* As my mind was racing, I picked up a copy of *Today's Parent* magazine and showed Sarah a list of fun activities we could do together during summer break. She pointed to a girl playing on the beach and told me she wanted to go swimming and build sandcastles.

When my name was called, a man in a white lab coat with a hospital ID badge clipped to the pocket escorted us to a tiny cubicle with a scale. He measured my weight and height and jotted them down on a pre-transplant assessment form attached to his clipboard. Then Sarah and I followed the white-coat man to an examination room to await Dr. Renner.

I googled Dr. Renner prior to our first meeting, which is something many patients do when they are assigned a new doctor. In Ontario, doctors' credentials and practice restrictions are posted on the College of Physicians and Surgeons of Ontario website. Dr. Renner's file confirmed what I'd suspected, that he is in an excellent transplant doctor with years of transplant experience.

During my appointment, Dr. Renner asked me several questions pertaining to risk factors for chronic liver disease: Did I have tattoos? Had I ever done illegal drugs? Did I drink alcohol? Did I smoke? Had I ever had a blood transfusion? Had I ever been on hemodialysis? The only question I answered yes to was the one about alcohol consumption. I said, "Maybe five drinks a year, more when I was a student. "

After a thorough physical exam, I sat back down on the chair next to the desk and watched Dr. Renner type his physical findings. Sarah snuggled up next to me and placed her head on my lap while sniffing the ear of her bunny blanket. She was used to accompanying me to doctors' appointments and was always shy and quiet.

Dr. Renner discussed the pre-transplant evaluation process, provided surgical details, and explained long-term post-transplant management. He explained I would be on anti-rejection medications for life. He answered all the questions I had written in my journal, taking away some of the fears I had about transplantation.

Dr. Renner explained how a patient is placed on the transplant waiting list. MELD (Model for End-Stage Liver Disease) is the scoring system used to assess the severity of chronic liver disease. It is useful in determining prognosis and prioritization for receipt of a liver transplant. MELD uses blood test results for bilirubin, creatinine, and the international normalized ratio (INR) for prothombin time. Bilirubin is high in patients who are jaundiced (yellow-coloured). Creatinine is high when kidney function is poor. INR is high when blood takes a long time to clot. Basically, the higher the MELD score, the sicker the patient. The sicker the patient, the higher that patient's placement on the transplant waiting list.

Any patients with a MELD score of fifteen or higher would benefit from a liver transplant to improve their health and prolong their life. My MELD score that day was, according to Dr. Renner's notes, "at least fifteen."

We discussed the option of a living donor, to shorten the time I would have to wait for a deceased donor liver. I said that I would try to find a family member or friend willing to voluntarily donate a portion of his or her liver.

We also spoke of the possibility of me developing insulin-dependent diabetes post-transplant. Corticosteroids (prednisone) and tacrolimus taken post-transplant, coupled with a history of gestational diabetes, increases the risk of developing diabetes. Given my lifelong needle phobia, I couldn't imagine poking myself with an insulin needle several times a day.

And so began the official pre-transplant work-up . . .

The pre-transplant work-up included a battery of medical tests to provide a complete story of my overall health and determine that I was a suitable transplant candidate. If there was something else wrong with me, the doctors were going to find out. The tests try to ensure that a patient can tolerate the physical and emotional stresses of surgery and the gruelling post-operative recovery period.

The computed tomography (CT) scan of my abdomen showed detailed images of my liver and its blood vessels, and other organs and structures such as lymph nodes, and also screened for liver cancer. The magnetic resonance imaging (MRI) scan provided detailed pictures of my abdominal organs and other structures inside my body. Both imaging tests were scheduled back-to-back late one Thursday night so I would only have to make one trip to Toronto. Having late-night testing mid-week had its advantages. Parking outside the Princess Margaret Hospital was free and traffic was light.

I had several abdominal ultrasounds taken. Some (to assess gallstones and estimate the amount of fluid in my abdomen) were done at St. Mary's Hospital because it was convenient for me to go the medical imaging department while on break.

The medical imaging tests revealed that I had a significantly enlarged spleen, measuring about twenty-four centimetres in length (a normal spleen measures seven to fourteen centimetres). The splenic vein appeared enlarged with a 5.3-centimeter blood clot. There were mobile gallstones and gallbladder wall thickening consistent with cholecystitis (gallbladder inflammation). There was a moderate amount of ascites in my abdomen and pelvis. There was normal blood flow through the portal and hepatic veins. My pancreas, bladder, and both kidneys appeared normal. *At least something appeared normal in my body.*

Several chest X-rays were taken to screen for any possible lung disorders (such as pneumonia), heart disorders (such as an enlarged heart), or fractured bones, including the ribs and collarbone. Nothing significant was noted on my X-rays.

A bone density scan was taken because I have a smaller body frame and had been taking prednisone since I was thirteen-years-old. The bone density scan is part of the work-up because there is a risk for fractures during and after surgery if a patient has low bone density. The bone density scan indicated that I had decreased bone mineralization consistent with the diagnosis of osteopenia. The bone density report did, however, state that my bone density showed no further worsening compared to the last scan back in 2006.

Pulmonary function tests (PFTs) were conducted to check how well my lungs worked. My report showed my lungs were normal and healthy with good lung capacity.

Comprehensive blood work is an essential piece in the transplant work-up, and, of course, one of my most feared medical tests. The lab technician drew twenty-one, ten-millilitre tubes of blood. *I kid you not!* I counted each tube as she placed them in a row on her desk. In addition to being tested for everything from organ function to viral infection, my blood was also typed and screened for antibodies so that blood would be available for transfusion during surgery.

The technician who drew my blood also performed an electrocardiogram (EKG). The EKG is used to identify heart rhythm concerns. While lying on a hard table in a cluttered room in the back of the lab, I was plastered with white, sticky buttons. Colourful wires were snapped to the buttons and produced a recording of my heart's electrical activity, including heart rate. The technician tore the EKG paper recording from the machine's printer and placed it in a manila folder. I asked if I could see my EKG. She handed me the recording and I said, "Yep, I'm in a normal sinus rhythm with a heart rate of sixty-four beats per minute." She smiled and commented that I must work in cardiology.

I also had an echocardiogram, which is an ultrasound of the heart. An echocardiogram shows how well the heart is pumping, examines the heart valves, and estimates the blood pressure in different parts of the heart. It is performed by lightly moving a probe across the skin that delivers sound waves to produce an image of the heart on a computer screen. Echocardiogram results provide insight into whether the heart can withstand a liver transplant, and whether additional cardiac testing is necessary. My cardiac work-up showed no cardiac anomalies. *I've always been told I have a good heart!*

A liver biopsy is also usually completed pre-op. However, I had had a liver biopsy one year ago while hospitalized at St. Mary's, so another procedure was not needed.

Now all that was left was for my case to be discussed at a liver transplant listing meeting. A team of doctors would review my pre-transplant test results, health status, and any issues that could disqualify me for surgery. If I were deemed a suitable candidate for transplant, I would be added to the liver transplant waiting list, with my placement on the list determined by my MELD score. If my condition changed after being listed, my MELD score would be reassessed and my position on the waiting list would change accordingly.

Dr. Renner had assessed my MELD score as "at least fifteen" on June 25. Little did Dr. Renner or I know that, in less than a month, my MELD score would rapidly increase from fifteen to forty-one.

Chapter 9

CHANGING ROLES

In the months prior to my transplant, I had felt changes in my body that suggested my liver disease was worsening, and that I was once again heading toward changing roles from nurse to patient. When I moved, I could feel fluid sloshing around inside my swollen abdomen. The extra fluid and my enlarged spleen pushed on my belly button and caused it to protrude outward. I wore a pregnancy belt to help push my belly button inward and alleviate some of the abdominal pain the umbilical hernia was causing. I was tired of telling patients who inquired about my due date, "I'm not pregnant, I have a liver disease."

After a twelve-hour shift, my ankles and feet were swollen to the point my shoes were tight. I wore knee-high compression stockings to help keep fluid out of my lower extremities. I have had problems with my feet since living in the Netherlands. I still blame all those years of walking on cobblestone streets and on the hard concrete floors in our Dutch house. Whatever the cause, I have endured years of suffering from heel pain due to plantar fasciitis. The condition had even caused me to be casted and wheelchair-bound for six weeks while we were living in the Netherlands. Unfortunately, the added fluid weight gain and swelling in my legs and feet exacerbated the plantar fasciitis, as did walking on the concrete floors in the hospital. I managed my heel pain with custom orthotics and proper running shoes, and with effective but torturous high-frequency ultrasound shock wave therapy, but it became so agonizing that when I climbed out of bed in the mornings, I had to crawl to the bathroom and stretch my calves while brushing my teeth.

Some weeks, my gallstones didn't bother me. Other weeks, they caused multiple episodes of excruciating pain that could last up to six hours and required morphine to deal with.

It had been years since I had had to deal with a prolapsed uterus, but with the extra fluid in my abdomen putting pressure on my already weak pelvic muscles, I wasn't happy when I had to begin wearing my pessary again to keep my uterus in place. My periods also stopped for six months during this time. This was something I didn't mind, and I saved money on feminine hygiene products.

I was becoming increasingly fatigued and needed to nap more. I napped during all my half-hour breaks at work. On my days off work, I took a three-hour nap while the kids were at school. On the days when Sarah was home with me, I still slept, but I put the TV "babysitter" on and told her to only wake me up if there was an emergency, which worked fine, except on days like the one on which she snooped through my makeup case and applied mascara as lipstick and lipstick on her eyebrows. She asked me, "Mommy, do I look pretty?" Of course she looked pretty. I didn't get upset with her, how could I? *Next time ask Mommy for a makeup lesson.*

My jaundiced colour frightened some of my patients. One female patient in particular stands out. I was sitting on her bed, teaching her about medications and reviewing her angiogram results. She listened intently, but I could sense she was curious about my colour. I don't always share my disease with patients, but I told her I had a liver disease and would someday need a liver transplant. When I came back into her room to administer her noon meds, she pulled back her blankets and offered me her bed. "You look sicker than me, my dear. How about you have a nap, I won't tell anyone." During my last week at work, the yellowing of my eyes and skin became so prominent that it frightened not only some of the patients but some of the nurses as well. They knew that no matter how many times I said I was fine, I wasn't.

My family and I noticed I was starting to become confused. One of the liver's jobs is to change toxic substances that are either made by the body or taken into the body (such as medicine and alcohol) into harmless ones. When the liver is damaged, like mine was, toxins, including ammonia, build up in the bloodstream. The build-up of ammonia can damage the nervous system and lead to a condition of decreased brain function called hepatic encephalopathy, the results of which can range from mild confusion to coma and brain death. Thankfully, my hepatic encephalopathy caused only forgetfulness and confusion, which were bad enough.

I usually have a good memory, but now I caught myself forgetting and confusing the simplest of things. I sent Kyle to school with princess lunch containers (on more than one occasion), which is embarrassing for an eight-year-old boy. I forgot that I had biked to Sobeys grocery store and went looking for my car in the parking lot. I made a cup of tea and put orange juice instead of milk in my mug. I got into the car one day and couldn't remember how to start it.

I was also having trouble remembering simple tasks at work. Once I even forgot to take out an IV upon discharge. The patient was ready to leave with his wife and daughter. He had all his belongings packed and said his goodbyes to staff. When he turned around to shake my hand and thank me for his care, I noticed he still had his IV in his right forearm. These are things I just don't forget!

I became more irritable, particularly at home. I was short with my husband and would yell at him for no reason. If he didn't do the dishes just so or left crumbs on the counter, I flipped out and told him off. I quickly lost my temper with the kids too. I found myself saying and doing things to the kids that didn't make any sense. When Sarah didn't approve of the clothes I picked out for her to wear to school and took time to find a different outfit, I became so angry that I swore at her and threw clothes at her. This is not my personality. I was a monster. I still feel bad that I hurt my family. I had so much rage inside. I became a complete stranger to my family and myself.

My blood sugars, for some unknown reason, started to plummet during the mornings. These hypoglycemic episodes caused me to feel jittery, faint, tired, and nauseated. At work I had to go against the ban on having food and drink in patient care areas and keep a Ziploc bag of digestive cookies and Smarties in my nursing scrub jacket pocket because I didn't have time to take a break, but I needed to take care of myself so I could continue taking care of patients. My family doctor, Dr. Winter, referred me to an endocrinologist, who wanted to test me for diabetes, but I was transplanted before I had a chance to complete the tests.

Everything I ate seemed to go straight through me. At home, I didn't stray far from the bathroom and found myself there as many as twenty times a day. When I needed to go to work or go out, I didn't eat much, just in case. In addition, my hemorrhoids were painful and itchy and sometimes bled. These problems were embarrassing and I just really wanted them to go away.

My body could only take so much. I often caught myself thinking, *Oh, how I envy healthy people; they have nothing to complain about.* Once, when Sarah had a teeny-tiny cut on her index finger (even *she* had to find it to point it out), and tears were pouring down her face like her finger was going to fall off, I put a Band-Aid on her finger and bingo, of course, she was instantly better. I wished I could have put a Band-Aid on my problems and been instantly better too.

I don't know how I managed to work with a failing liver those last few months. I should have called in sick on several occasions, but being a nurse and a mother, I am used to being the caretaker and am stubborn and feel invincible at times. I was concerned about leaving my nursing co-workers short-staffed, taking care of patients, and making money. I didn't have my priorities straight, and I was in denial about the severity of my condition. *I'm fine . . . this is just another flare-up . . . I need more prednisone and then I'll be good to go again.* But I wasn't fine, and I wasn't good to go.

The visit to the pre-transplant clinic on June 25 had shed some light on the situation; a liver transplant would hopefully "cure" all my ailments. But that was something that was going to happen in the future, not something that was going to happen immediately. I didn't have much choice but to continue on with life as I knew it: making frequent trips to the bathroom, eating very little, wearing a pregnancy belt, napping. My life continued on for a couple weeks longer before I crashed.

It was summer holidays for Kyle and Sarah, so we went to Belleville for the first weekend in July. Friends and family commented on how terrible I looked—jaundiced and fluid-filled. Mom, the kids, and I spent a day at my grandparents' farm. Instead of playing outside with the kids, picking berries and building a fort with the hay bales, I spent all afternoon sleeping on the couch. I was tired of being tired, and felt I was spending more time asleep than awake. Life was passing me by.

My last shift, on Monday, July 8, I was scheduled for twelve hours but only managed to complete eight. I was caring for one of our frequent-flyer heart failure patients and helped him up to a chair for lunch. In a heavy Lithuanian accent, he told me I should go home. I literally couldn't function anymore and sat on the foot of his bed and rested my head on the footboard. The patient didn't say anything; he let me rest. I kept thinking, *I can't go on like this . . . I'm so sick and miserable . . . I want to go home to bed.*

One of my co-workers offered to help me when she found me resting on my patient's bed. I was so grateful when she finished getting my patients out of bed for lunch, checked their blood sugars, and set up their tray tables. I informed our charge nurse that I needed to go home. My co-workers were all well informed of my condition and had watched as my health had slowly deteriorated. There was no problem with me ending my shift early, but there was a problem with the fact that I had my bike at work and my body wouldn't allow me to make the five-kilometer jaunt home.

Usually, the only time I don't bike the five kilometers each way to and from work is when there's snow or ice on the ground, or when there's a thunderstorm. It doesn't take any longer to cycle than to drive by the time I park and walk from the parking lot to the hospital. Kevin and I knew there was a problem when I started calling him after shifts, asking him to pick me up—I never did that before. Once home, I would shower and go straight to bed. Kyle and Sarah stayed up later than I did. It became the norm for *them* to tuck *me* in and read me stories.

I contacted Dr. Shah that same day because the ascites was worsening. I had a water-baby inside. He scheduled me for a paracentesis, or abdominal tap, appointment the next day, to remove some of the fluid from my abdominal cavity. Of course, I cringe every time I think of this procedure because it involves some really big needles. I tried to focus on the positive side—the relief I would feel in my abdomen after the fluid was drained.

Dr. Shah "tapped" me the next day, Tuesday, July 9. I like to think that I was tapped much like a maple tree. Only the fluid isn't sweet and clear like sap. My ascites fluid during this tap looked like pale yellow urine. It took an hour to drain 1.5 litres of fluid from my abdomen. Dr. Shah was hoping for a little more, but the catheter accidentally pulled out while he was absent from the room. I didn't panic, but instead became my own nurse and finished taking it out myself, then put pressure over the site and a light dressing.

After the tap, I had my blood tested at the hospital lab. I had been on monthly lab draws, so Dr. Shah kept a close eye on my liver function. The lab draw revealed that my liver enzymes were elevated, as we had expected. Two of my liver enzymes, AST and ALT, had climbed considerably: AST 336 (normal is 5 to 40 U/L) and ALT 386 (normal is 24 to 57 U/L). My INR was high at 2.9 (0.9 to 1.2 is normal), and platelets were markedly decreased at nineteen (normal is 150 to 400). Having such high INR and low platelets meant I was having blood clotting issues and bruised even more easily than usual. I was black and blue from building a pergola in our backyard. Every time I knelt down on the wood to paint, my knees bruised. When I carried the wood from our garage to the backyard, my arms bruised. Yes, I was busy sanding wood, painting, and assembling a pergola while I was sick. I really wanted the project completed so I would have a backyard swing and place to retreat to in the summer.

The tap left my abdomen feeling sore where the catheter had been, and I was experiencing some stomach cramping. I only made it two blocks down the road from Toronto Western Hospital before I knew I needed to find a toilet. Finding a public bathroom in downtown Toronto is a quest in itself. There is nowhere to park outside most restaurants and businesses, and many require you to be a customer to use their facilities. Luckily I stumbled upon a port-a-potty in a nearby park. The port-a-potty was sitting in a big puddle of water because it was two days after the big Toronto flood of 2013. I got a soaker as I stepped into the port-a-potty. Of course, there was no toilet paper. Luckily again, I had a few crumpled tissues in my purse.

I made it as far as Mississauga (in other words, not very far) before I had to stop again, this time at a Tim Hortons. When I looked in the mirror in the bathroom, I noticed that my cheeks were flushed. I felt my forehead. I was burning up. I splashed some cool water on my face and stood in the bathroom under the air conditioning vent. My abdomen began cramping badly, and I was buckled over in pain. I didn't have any other choice but to try to drive home. Kevin couldn't come to my rescue because I had the car. I climbed back into the driver's seat and turned just in time to vomit onto the pavement. I was so sick, so very sick! It felt like my body was giving up; my liver disease was going to kill me right then and there. I rolled down the window and slept in the parking lot for over an hour, then made my way home. When I arrived home, I took my temperature. Yes, I was fevered—39.8 degrees Celsius to be exact.

I received a call from Dr. Shah early the next morning, Wednesday, July 10. He informed me I had an infection in the fluid in my abdomen. I was still fevered, at forty degrees Celsius. The organism causing the infection had not yet been identified, as it takes a few days to grow the culture. But confirmation of an infection meant I needed something a little more potent than the oral antibiotics I was taking, and Dr. Shah advised me to go to the emergency department for antibiotic therapy.

I rushed around the house and collected some belongings, with the presumption I was going to be admitted, shoved them into my old UVic backpack, and then raided the cupboards for food. Since I am a picky eater and hospital food isn't the most appealing, I always pack food.

After Kevin checked me into the emergency room, he left and drove to work. Normally, when one takes a family member to the ER, one stays with said family member. However, this was my place of employment, so Kevin knew I would be in good hands. He also knew from past experience that I was going to be there awhile, and there wouldn't have been anything he could do but watch and wait. I called him frequently with updates. *Hi Kevin, I'm lying here with IV antibiotics, nothing exciting, I keep dozing in and out of sleep, still waiting for a bed on the floor.* Four hours later . . . *Hi Kevin, nope, I don't have a bed yet, but I was given a supper tray that came with rice pudding.* Four more hours later . . . *Hi Kevin, I don't think I'm ever going to get a bed, and lying on this inch-thin mattress is killing my back.*

A resident doctor took my health history and performed a thorough physical exam. The plan was to administer a five-day course of IV antibiotics. The first dose was infused in the ER while I waited for a bed on the floor.

After returning home from visiting me that evening—and finding me in the same place he'd left me ten hours earlier—Kevin phoned family to let them know I was in the hospital and had an infection. I didn't know it then, but Kevin later told me, "When

I took you to the hospital this time, I had a gut feeling there was a real possibility that this could be the time where you went into the hospital and didn't come out alive."

Word spread among family and friends that I was in the hospital. My brother Andy called my brother Bill and informed him that he should get tested, as he might be a possible living donor (more on that in chapter fourteen).

The nurse-patient relationship is one that I am extremely familiar with from both sides of the bed. It was surreal that on Monday I'd worked as a nurse and on Wednesday I was admitted as a patient. I wanted to be placed on our inpatient cardiology floor again because I liked having my co-workers care for me, but there were no beds available.

I was admitted to a semi-private room on the fifth floor, the general medicine department. My roommate was in the process of being discharged, which meant I didn't have anyone beside me that night. That's the thing about a semi-private room, you never know who you are going to bunk with. I've had patients share a room who became such good friends that they exchanged phone numbers after their stay. Then I've had patients share a room who had to be moved so there wouldn't be trouble. Once, a young female patient was so obnoxious to her roommate that the roommate, a middle-aged woman, threw pillows at her and told her to shut up and not act so rude.

My nurse completed the admission assessment. She asked me questions about my health history and completed the usual head-to-toe assessment. She told me I made her admission assessment easy because I answered her questions without prompting and used medical terms to describe my health. If my nurse had given me the computer, I could have entered my own admission assessment data.

Dr. Golubov was assigned to my case. I knew Dr. Golubov because he is one of the gastroenterologists who frequents our unit when we have the occasional gastrointestinal patient. He is the go-to doctor for anything stomach- and bowel-related. Dr. Golubov explained that my peritoneal fluid was positive for the bacterium E. Coli. *Well, that explains my digestive problems.* I don't know how I contracted the infection, but I speculate that it may have been while caring for a female patient who had similar symptoms. I did wear gloves and practise proper handwashing after having contact with her, but with my suppressed immune system it doesn't take much to get me sick.

I was continued on the antibiotic ceftriaxone to treat the infection, but the dose was decreased from two grams to one gram because ceftriaxone can lead to severe kidney and liver impairment, and my sick liver was already having issues.

My peritoneal fluid was infected with E. coli, so the question was, was E. coli present in other areas of my body? Samples were taken to find out. The test results were alarming. I had E. coli not only in my peritoneal fluid, but also in my blood, urine, and stool. I was a walking infection!

The only good thing about having an infection was being assigned to a private room. Mind you, I was stuck in isolation, but I didn't have to share my space with a complete stranger. Being in isolation meant all visitors and staff had to don a yellow isolation gown and wear gloves. When I wanted to leave my room, I had to don a yellow gown and gloves as well. When I wandered the halls dressed in isolation garb, I felt all eyes were on me. *Pssst . . . Stay away from her, she's got an infection.*

The decidedly unpleasant symptoms of my infection subsided, but I was kept in the hospital after finishing the five-day course of IV antibiotics because my abdominal fluid had returned and my liver enzymes, which had already been elevated well beyond the normal range, had increased significantly. In addition to continuing my daily dosages of Imuran and prednisone, Dr. Golubov also prescribed Lasix and Aldactone to help rid my body of the excess fluid. My kidneys were still functioning well, so I was able to make good use of these diuretics.

Dr. Golubov and I knew my condition was deteriorating. Every day, my liver enzymes increased and my INR and platelets showed that my body was having trouble clotting its blood. After lab draws, I had to keep the cotton ball on my arm and apply at least ten minutes of pressure to stop the bleeding. I was given a vitamin K injection to help improve blood clotting.

The other thing that happened was that due to my hepatic encephalopathy, I became increasingly confused. Kevin later told me I sounded like a babbling idiot when speaking with him on the phone. He said that sometimes I would say something, and then end up contradicting myself by the end of the conversation, that speaking with me reminded him of when he was young and spent time with his nana, who had Alzheimer's.

I found that sometimes, my mind was clear and I could sit and have a perfectly coherent conversation with visitors. Other times, my brain was in a fog. I even had difficulty managing a simple task like taking a shower. I had trouble applying body wash onto the washcloth and forgot to wash the cream rinse out of my hair.

While I was hospitalized, Kevin was back at it, dealing with sick me and managing the kids and the household while working full-time. He had to do the things I normally do. I can only imagine how he dealt with Sarah's long, tangled hair or made sure Kyle bathed himself. It was difficult for Kevin to keep it all together on the home front with the kids on summer break, but since I had a chronic condition and had spent extended periods of time in the hospital, it was nothing he hadn't done before.

Mom took some time off work and drove to Kitchener on Thursday, July 11. She wanted to be with her daughter, and she helped Kevin hold down the fort in my absence. Kevin and mom continually brought me things like new underwear, reading material, my Nintendo DS video games, and, of course, food. I sometimes felt they were my hospital mules. They always kept me well stocked. Mom often brought treats when she visited, like Dairy Queen strawberry milkshakes.

During my hospitalization, many of my co-workers visited me as well, or I sometimes trekked down to 3 East to visit them. It was an excuse to go for a walk. I remember all the nurse practitioners sitting in my room to find out how I was faring. They offered help with the kids and to make meals. My co-workers were incredibly supportive, and I am tremendously thankful to them. It was comforting to know I have so many wonderful friends willing to help my family during a difficult time.

One of St. Mary's chaplains, Cindy, provided much-needed spiritual support. Cindy came to my room and stood at my bedside. She held my hands, we closed our eyes, and she calmly and quietly said a prayer of healing for the sick. I'm not an overly religious person, but I felt comforted by her prayer and blessing. It was like a weight was lifted off my shoulders, and I felt reassured knowing that I would have God watching over me as I made my transplant journey.

I was given a day pass from St. Mary's on Friday, July 12, to attend some of my mandatory pre-transplant work-up appointments (bone density scan, chest X-ray, and pulmonary function tests) at Princess Margaret Hospital in Toronto. When Kevin returned me to St. Mary's, I didn't want to exit the car. I wanted him to keep driving to our house. I felt like I was doing jail time.

Dr. Golubov was well aware of my need for a liver transplant. He and I both knew I needed to be transferred to the Toronto General Hospital (TGH) transplant unit *now*. The frustrating problem was, there were no beds available in the inpatient transplant unit. I was basically in a holding pattern. I was becoming sicker by the day, yet I had no place to go. Dr. Golubov was in constant contact with the transplant team in Toronto. He was worried and tried his best to get me transferred sooner. I asked him if my husband and mom could drive me to Toronto and take me to the ER at TGH and force the hospital to admit me. Would that secure a bed for me sooner?

Given my condition at this point, I have to rely on my husband to fill in some gaps.

"Christine went into the hospital at a MELD score of eighteen on Wednesday, July 10, and by Sunday, July 14, she had a MELD of twenty-four [if you remember from the last chapter, a MELD score of fifteen or higher means a person is a good candidate for transplant]. Christine's mom and I kept thinking, 'If they don't transfer her soon, she is going to die first.' The other thing that scared us is that she needed a new liver, but she wasn't on the transplant waiting list yet. You can't get a new liver if you aren't on the list, and she hadn't completed the screening process despite our trip to Princess Margaret Hospital on July 12. The transplant team didn't even know she needed a new liver!

"It is my opinion that if TGH could have seen Christine's lab results, she would have been transferred two days earlier. St. Mary's and TGH don't share a computer information system—if they did, TGH would have noticed there was a serious problem. St. Mary's was sending Christine's lab updates by fax, but her condition deteriorated so quickly that the information system updates just didn't happen as fast as they needed to."

I remember talking to Kevin on the phone the evening before I was transferred. It was clear to Kevin and my mom that no matter what the hospital said, Kevin was going to take me to the emergency department at TGH. Kevin was freaking out. He was afraid he was going to lose me if I didn't get a new liver right away—I was quickly fading. He had never seen me so sick in all of our twenty years together. On Wednesday, July 17, though he couldn't say it out loud for liability reasons, I felt like Dr. Golubov was considering letting me sign out AMA (Against Medical Advice) so my family could drive me to TGH.

Thankfully, that day, and a week after I was admitted to St. Mary's, a bed opened up on the seventh-floor inpatient transplant unit at TGH, and I prepared to be sent to there by ambulance.

Chapter 10

LISTED

The paramedics transferring me to Toronto General Hospital wheeled a stretcher into my room, belted me onto it, and covered me with a crisp, white sheet. I was not looking forward to the ambulance ride since I have a really big problem with motion sickness— *the Jowett stomach* was about to strike again.

We had not even made it to the ambulance and I could already feel my stomach churning. The quick turns through the hallways, and the fact I was being wheeled on the stretcher, were making me queasy. The dose of Gravol my nurse had given me half an hour before the transfer didn't seem to be helping. The stretcher ride was as bad as the Tilt-a-Whirl ride at the fair, something I hadn't gone on since I was a kid. And like at an amusement park, I kept all my hands and feet "inside the ride," folded safely on the stretcher as instructed, as I was loaded into the ambulance—wouldn't want to lose a limb in the transfer.

The ambulance was equipped with everything medical. It was kind of neat looking around at all the knobs and tubing and drawers labelled with drugs and equipment. *A mini emergency room on wheels.* Kevin sat in the passenger seat in the front of the ambulance. Before we left, I asked if I could sit facing forward, looking out the tiny window between the back and the cab. The paramedic next to me in the back said it was policy that patients remain strapped to the stretcher. *Policies, shmolicies! The person who wrote that policy must not get motion sick.*

And get motion sick I did. Anyone who's ever taken a ride in the back of an ambulance knows that the windows are obscured so you can't see out. This, combined with the fact I was facing backwards and that the ambulance rocked and rolled as we went around corners, was a recipe for disaster. Even when there was nothing left in my stomach, I continued to retch

The paramedic felt really sorry for me. She placed a cool, wet cloth on my forehead. She rubbed my back. She was so calm and genuinely tried to comfort me. I felt bad that she felt bad, and I was afraid I was going to make everyone else in the ambulance sick. The paramedics knew I wasn't going to survive the ambulance ride to Toronto. We had only made it about ten minutes down the road, and I hadn't stopped using my barf bag. The paramedics decided to make an exception to their policy on the patient being strapped to a stretcher. They made a pit stop to unstrap me from the stretcher and belt me into the "jump seat" instead. The jump seat is a little seat in the back of the ambulance that, to my relief, faced forward so I could look through the tiny window and watch the road. The paramedic strapped herself into a seat beside me. She sat sideways and could not see out. I asked her if she ever gets motion sick, and she said she was glad she was not prone to motion sickness because she couldn't imagine doing this job while feeling nauseous. The paramedic offered me mint-flavoured gum, which I happily accepted.

I kept my eyes on the road while aggressively chewing my gum. We got to Toronto before rush-hour traffic. I asked the paramedic what would happen if we got stuck in a traffic jam, and she said that we would put the lights on and move past the traffic. I was glad we didn't have to speed along; the ride was bumpy enough. But then again, it would have been fun to swerve around other cars with the sirens wailing and lights flashing. *Get out of the way, people, this is an emergency, my liver is about to blow.*

The paramedic had kept a close eye on me and occasionally asked how I was doing. I was queasy the entire trip, but once I could see out, I wasn't sick again—that is until we made a couple of sharp turns during the final stretch of our trip through the city. Between bouts of vomiting, I glanced at the paramedic with my sick, jaundiced eyes and mustered, "Are we there yet?" I had never felt so grateful to see another hospital as I did when we pulled up outside the ER of TGH and I was able to set foot onto solid ground. I haven't seen the paramedics again since that day, but I'm hoping our paths cross again, perhaps during one of my patients' transfers or in passing in the St. Mary's hospital lobby, so I can thank them for helping me survive the trip to Toronto. I'm certain they will remember me.

Kevin helped settle me into my new room, a semi-private with a window looking out toward several hospital buildings. At least I finally had a bed and didn't die waiting for one to become available. The nurse checked me in and performed a set of vitals—blood pressure, temperature, heart rate, respiratory rate. A doctor came in shortly after and did an assessment and ordered blood work. She probed me with questions about what was going on while reviewing the stack of my medical records we had brought with us in the transfer. Periodically during this conversation, I would be talking with the doctor and then "check out," as Kevin put it. I would nod off for about ten seconds, and then wake up and continue the conversation like nothing had happened. It was like I needed to take a short nap, but was hyper-aware of my surroundings. I knew I was "checking out" but I couldn't control it. The doctor noted this narcoleptic-type symptom, but she didn't seem too concerned.

Kevin departed around 8:30 p.m. to make it to the Greyhound bus terminal in time to catch a bus back to Kitchener. Mom was still at our house and was taking care of Kyle and Sarah, which had given Kevin the opportunity to make the trip with me to Toronto. Mom's help was a godsend. I needed Kevin's support. I needed him with me, even if that just meant having him present to ease my fears and anxieties. I was unsure of what to expect during the ambulance transfer (Was I going to die en route, since it felt like I vomited up my guts?) or once I made it to the transplant unit (Was I going to be transplanted that night? Was I going to get sicker and end up in the ICU?).

Kevin left me, but I wasn't alone because I had a roommate. She was a new heart-transplant recipient. She kept to herself because she was very sick and having difficulty breathing. I could hear her wheezing and hyperventilating. It was so tempting to pull back the curtains and give her supplemental oxygen, but she was in isolation. Her side of the room was curtained off, and anyone who entered her space had to don the usual isolation gown and gloves and, in her case, a facemask. I had to avoid her because I didn't need to complicate my problems with another infection. I wanted to say something to her through the curtains, but I knew striking up a conversation would make it that much harder for her to breathe. Since my roommate was hidden behind curtain number one, she was given a bedside commode and had her own sink so she wouldn't contaminate our shared bathroom. This meant I had the bathroom to myself.

My roommate kept me up all night. When I dozed off, I would wake to the noise of her laboured and gasping breathing, or to her calling her nurse in to help with this, that, and the other thing. So the next day, Thursday, July 18, I was *very* tired. I don't remember much about the morning because I slept after I ate breakfast. Even when my childhood friend Sue stopped by to visit and leave me some magazines and crossword puzzles, I continued to sleep. Sue didn't wake me because she told me I looked like I was peacefully sleeping. I also slept through lunch, but it didn't matter because I couldn't eat what I found beside me on my lunch tray when I awoke anyway—cold mystery meat and a stale bun. I had money tucked away in my blue UVic backpack, so I slipped down to the Starbucks on the first floor for a grande chai tea and a blueberry bar instead.

Sometime in the afternoon, my roommate was moved to a private isolation room. I felt so bad for her; she had just been through a complicated heart transplant surgery, and now she had to deal with a life-threatening infection. The only thing I learned from her was she had acquired some type of bacterial pneumonia lung infection for which she required potent antibiotic therapy, and that the antibiotics had to be approved by the Ministry of Health in Ottawa because they were expensive and she required a thirty-day treatment regimen. I knew the other bed in my room would be filled quickly because the inpatient transplant unit is a busy place, a revolving door of sick patients waiting for a transplant, of patients recovering from a transplant, and of living donors.

The afternoon was a little blurry to me. I was sick and not thinking straight, and that, combined with the lack of sleep the night before, made my mind foggy. I often caught myself doing and saying some weird things. I somehow managed to wander into the medication dispensing room during one of my walks. *Maybe I thought I was working that day.* People I didn't know (I'm assuming they were nurses because they wore royal blue TGH hospital scrubs) routinely went into and out of my room. One of these people tested my blood, and another took me for a chest X-ray. I just went with the flow of things.

I still had not completed the entire pre-transplant process and was not on the transplant list yet. The next step was a meeting with the social worker, Sonali. She spent some time with me in the afternoon, reviewing important details like drug coverage, finances, and family support. She left me a post-liver-transplant manual, which answered many questions I had about liver transplantation. There was a section on complications encountered in the early post-transplant period: diabetes, wound infection, internal bleeding. I only read a snippet of it because I didn't want to know what *could* happen. The manual also explained which medications I would take post-transplant, a little about the ICU stay, and care after discharge.

It was like my pregnancy bible, except it was *What to Expect When You're Expecting a Liver Transplant.*

Dr. Lilly and other members of the liver transplant team stopped by my room around suppertime. This was the first time I met Dr. Lilly, a tall, slender man with glasses and a scruffy beard, and a long, white lab jacket with his hospital ID badge dangling from the chest pocket. I instantly liked him; he was kind, personable, and knowledgeable, and he took the time to talk with me. He explained how a liver transplant listing meeting is conducted and what would be discussed—my sick liver and me. The team reviews the patient's pre-transplant test results, health history, current blood tests, and MELD score. They also look at any contraindications—anything that would preclude the patient from having surgery, or anything that could complicate recovery. Dr. Lilly explained that the team would be meeting tomorrow afternoon to review my case for the transplant waiting list. He promised to stop by after the meeting and inform me of the outcome.

On Thursday afternoon Mom stopped by for a brief visit on her way back home to Belleville. She restocked my food supplies and brought new pajamas and underwear. She also told me my aunt Margi and cousin Amy wanted to set up phone service in my room so it would be easier to get in touch with me. I was moved that my family was looking out for me by thinking of little things like that. Kevin had left me the computer, so I was also able to email updates to friends and family and post updates on Facebook.

I wasn't feeling particularly well when Mom was there. I was nauseated, and the "checking out" episodes were becoming more frequent. My body was tired and felt like it was fading. Plus I was nervous about the waiting list meeting the next day. I knew without a doubt I would be listed, but I was uncertain about my listing status. Would I be placed at the top of the list, or near the bottom? I also didn't know if I was still able to go the living-donor route and needed my cousin Catherine and brother to complete their living-donor evaluation process. All these unknowns were making me feel ill, and I couldn't focus on anything. This was my future that the transplant team was going to discuss, the difference between living and the very real possibility of dying.

The doctors had the transplant team meeting on Friday, July 19—Kevin's thirty-ninth birthday. *Kevin's birthday? I didn't get him anything, not even a cake . . . but how could I? I've been cooped up in the hospital for over a week. Maybe Sarah drew him a picture? Maybe Kyle made something for him from the items in the blue recycling bin?* As it turned out, his brother Wesley bought a cake and celebrated Kevin's birthday with him. Wesley lives in Edmonton, but he was on a business trip in Mississauga, which isn't too far from Kitchener. The kids gave Daddy a fishing pole thanks to Mom's help. Kevin isn't much of a fisherman, but the kids wanted to get Daddy a fishing pole so he could go fishing with them.

Dr. Lilly turned up late in the afternoon with the news that I was officially listed. At least now I had a chance to receive a new liver. The following are excerpts from Dr. Renner's meeting note to my hepatologist, Dr. Shah:

As you are aware, this thirty-nine-year-old lady is known for autoimmune hepatitis–related liver cirrhosis. She was first seen in our clinic on June 25 and she was discovered to have an acute flare of her hepatitis with jaundice. She has rapidly decompensated further despite increasing her prednisone dose . . . The patient is jaundiced, has ascites and muscle wasting, as well as a history of variceal bleed back in 2007. Her MELD score is thirty-four . . .

There is no doubt that the patient has serious indications for a liver transplant. She has completed her transplant work-up. This did not reveal any relevant co-morbidities or contraindications. She was therefore accepted on our liver transplant waiting list today . . . [M]ost likely the patient will have to stay in the hospital until her transplant, given her severe liver decompensation.

I knew I was sick and my liver was rapidly failing, but it really hit home when Dr. Lilly told me I was placed at the top of the liver transplant list for my blood type. I was relieved to find out I was listed, but I was shocked and absolutely scared to death over this news. My MELD score and symptoms revealed that my end-stage liver disease had progressed to the point that I was now the sickest liver disease patient in Ontario. I was to receive the first liver that became available and was a match. I may be competitive by nature and like to be at the top, but certainly not in this case. Being at the top meant I was going to die if a liver did not become available immediately.

I didn't know how much time I had left to live, but I knew now that death was imminent if I wasn't transplanted. After Dr. Lilly left my room, I cried. I cried because I was scared I was going to die and never see my family again. I cried because my children would grow up without their mom. I cried because I was going to leave my husband a widower with two young children. I cried because I hadn't finished living life.

I prayed that a liver would become available in time to save my life. People waiting for their life-saving organ have an unknown wait time. Some wait for months, others for years. But each of us waits, prays, and hopes that our health will not deteriorate to the point that our body gives up while we're waiting for a donor family to consent to donate their loved one's organs so we may receive our life-saving gift.

On the Trillium Gift of Life Network (TGLN) website, organ donation and waiting list stats for Ontario are posted for the public to view. I checked the website. I was one of sixty-four female patients waiting for a liver transplant in Ontario. I thought, *Which of us will die waiting?* My answer to myself was, *None of us.* Idealistic as it was, I had to remain optimistic that organs would become available in time to save not only my life, but the lives of all those listed.

It occurred to me that praying for a liver to become available meant a stranger needed to die. Family and friends would need to mourn the passing of their loved one. It upset me to think that I was waiting in my hospital bed on the seventh floor of Toronto General for someone to die so I could live. It felt so selfish, so very wrong, yet something I had no control over. My need for a donor liver was in no way going to *cause* someone to die. I was not in control of where my new liver would come from. The donor would die even if I didn't need his or her liver. It was an emotional time as I sat alone in my hospital bed uncovering these deep-rooted and unnerving thoughts and feelings.

That night I tried to sleep on my uncomfortable, rigid hospital bed and starchy white linens, but couldn't. My new roommate, Shelly, wasn't able to sleep either; her Lasix diuretic had kicked in and she was up to pee every ten minutes. We had to compete for the bathroom because I was still having my own, different kind of issue in that department.

Between trips to the bathroom, we had the opportunity to chat. Shelly shared her transplant story with me (which you can read in the "Others' Transplant Journeys" section at the end of the book). She is from Peterborough and waited nine years before receiving her new kidney. Polycystic kidney disease was the culprit behind her kidney failure. It was touching to learn she had named her new kidney "Grace." Shelly told me she had named her new kidney—or her "new friend for life," as she put it—Grace because "by the grace of the Lord, He picked me to have this wonderful gift."

I finally fell into a restless sleep shortly before midnight thanks to the Ativan that my nurse slipped me, but was awakened shortly before 6 a.m. for labs. *Such a cruel alarm clock, and one I can't hit the snooze button on.* A few minutes later, a young resident doctor with the transplant team strutted into my room and stood at the foot of my bed. He was grinning. *Is this a nervous grin, or a happy grin?* I couldn't tell. But then I learned he was the bearer of some wonderful news. A liver had become available. I was about to jump out of bed, red-eyed from crying, and kiss him on his cheek. Instead, I distinctly remember saying, "No way, really? Are you sure? I was just listed yesterday afternoon, that was quick." The plan was for surgery that day—Saturday, July 20— at 3:15 p.m. What he said took a second to register. In less than ten hours, I was going to be getting a new liver. I was in shock that a liver had become available so quickly. My prayers were answered!

The doctor told me it was a good thing a liver was available because my condition was deteriorating rapidly every day, and he didn't think I had much more time to live. *How much time? Weeks? Days? Hours?* I needed to know the answer, and asked, but the resident told me he was not inclined to say because he didn't have a crystal ball and could not give me an exact time frame. Besides, he added, what difference would it make if he told me I had one day left to live, or one week left to live? Would that have changed my mind about having surgery? *Well, no, but I like to cross off days on the calendar to count down important events . . . death being one of them.*

Of course, as soon as the doctor left, I was immediately on the phone with Kevin and my parents, who spread the astounding news. It was not a surprise to family and friends that I had been listed, because they knew how ill I had become. It was, however, a relief to them that a donor liver had become available so quickly. My family said they would come to see me off to the operating room, where that afternoon my life was scheduled to be transformed with a recycled liver.

Shortly after 7 a.m., my day nurse, Linda, bounced into my room, very chipper and eager to start her day. She informed me that she would be the one prepping me for surgery once she received the go-ahead from the transplant team. She performed a thorough head-to-toe assessment. My blood pressure was in my boots: 74/50. Linda wasn't too concerned because I would be given several litres of fluid during surgery.

I glanced at the clock near the nurses' station on my way to the bathroom. Eight hours and counting until I would be given the gift of life. *Hang on, liver, you can make it, don't fail me now.*

I thought I was fasting, but a breakfast tray was brought to me. Linda popped her head in to inform me that I could eat a light breakfast at 7:30 a.m. because I had a late surgery time slot. Orange juice, tea, ginger ale, and Honey Nut Cheerios. As I sat eating breakfast, I thought, *What if this is my last meal?* Maybe I could request my favourite foods—crab, raspberries, and chocolate—just in case I never got to eat again. Then that little voice inside my head said, *Snap out of it, Christine, you will be just fine and able to indulge in all your favourite foods again really soon.*

Linda posted a NPO (Nil Per Os) sign on the wall over my bed. It was official; I was banned from eating for the rest of the day. I spent the morning wandering the hallways, since walking helped clear my mind and pacified my nervousness. Sitting in my room made me tense and fidgety. I had already organized my stack of magazines and clothes into piles. Waiting for a life-saving organ transplant was like being a kid waiting for Christmas morning to arrive, with all the excitement and anticipation of what Santa will place under the tree. The same feelings flooded my body—I was excited and anxious for surgery, yet *very* frightened.

My family arrived in one big mass around 10:30 a.m., and I literally ran into them near the elevators. I had been wandering the hallways over and over, surely etching a path into the floor. Mom and Dad came to visit. Kevin, his brother Wesley, and Sarah and Kyle arrived. And I had surprise visitors: my brother Andy and his wife, Mandy. I asked where Bill was, but he had to work. Kevin and Mom tended to be regular visitors, but having everyone else visit reassured me that everything would be okay. I missed having Kyle and Sarah wrap their little arms around me, and it felt good to receive big hugs and kisses on the cheek from both kids.

When Mandy and Andy saw me, they were pretty shocked. Mandy, who is a prison nurse, later told me, "I wasn't prepared to see you that sick. We had just been to the beach together not that long before . . . [I]t was a huge decline from the person I saw playing in the sand... I couldn't believe you were still walking around in the hospital and even participating in your own care."

As much as I truly appreciated my family's visit, it was largely a blur. I was still regularly "checking out" and I felt confused and in a fog. I remember Mom sneaking me a gift in a bag to give to Sarah for her birthday, which was the next day. This gesture was so sweet, as I had not been able to choose a birthday gift for Sarah. Sarah's thank-you hug was a priceless memory I could take to the operating room, and I had to wipe away the tears when she whispered to me, "Mommy, I don't want you to stay in the hospital because you are going to miss my birthday party."

Everyone stayed in the visitors' lounge and gave Kevin and I time alone in my room. Kevin sat beside me while we discussed "my wishes." I was so focused on having a life-saving transplant that I had failed to plan for my funeral or think about cremation and the location of my potential grave. Young people aren't supposed to plan for death, and in my mind I just knew I wasn't going to die. Kevin and I had made our will with a lawyer prior to moving to the Netherlands, so Kevin knew I didn't want to remain on life support if there was no hope of recovery. I reaffirmed the wish indicated by my being a registered donor and told Kevin if an unforeseen medical complication occurred and I passed away during or after surgery, to please donate all organs and tissues. In the best-case scenario, one donor can save up to eight lives. I figured my liver and kidneys would be disqualified, so I was down to saving up to five lives. There were many patients waiting for a life-saving organ on the seventh floor of TGH alone.

But as Kevin and I discussed the very grim topic of death, I remember my foggy brain thinking, *Why are we discussing what should be done if I die? I'm not going to die at thirty-nine-years-old, there is way too much to do in life.* It just didn't feel like it was my time yet. My internal motto was, *I am going to stay strong and survive.*

Things were not going as planned because it was around 3:45 p.m., past the expected time of surgery. We knew something was up. Mom, Andy, and Mandy were in my room when the resident doctor came in and abruptly and matter-of-factly delivered the heartbreaking news that surgery was a "no go." The doctor assured us that I was still at the top of the list for my blood type.

All I could think was, *What do you mean, surgery is no go?* I couldn't fathom the idea that the donor liver was not suitable for transplant. Surprisingly, I didn't shed a tear, or say anything. I knew I had the transplant team of doctors and nurses behind me, taking care of me and keeping me alive during this difficult waiting period. I was confident another liver would become available when the time was right. The waiting game would continue.

The waiting game can be a difficult time. It can be lonely and cause a lot of anxiety. There can be disappointing "dress rehearsals" like the one I had just experienced. Some people wait a couple of weeks for a life-saving organ to become available, while others, like my friend Andrea, wait for years.

I had envisioned carrying a pager around in my day-to-day life, waiting for *the call*, but my body became too ill too fast. I was fortunate, in a way, because my wait was unusually short and the wait was in hospital, where I had the transplant team to care for me as my liver disease progressed each day. I had health care professionals to help keep me alive while I waited for the perfect liver.

Of course, we were all let down, but it was best that surgery was cancelled if the liver wasn't good enough. There was no point in receiving a new liver that wasn't going to make me better or that was going to cause additional complications in the future. Surgery would happen when the timing was perfect, we just knew it and felt it.

Chapter 11

'TWAS THE NIGHT
BEFORE SURGERY

My family left for the day after learning surgery was called off. I was tired from their visit, so I slept until 7:15 p.m., when the nurses' chatter loudened and woke me during shift change.

My night nurse entered my room and wrote her name on the whiteboard hanging on the wall. After she performed a set of vitals, she brought me a paper medicine cup containing my medications. I checked my dispensed meds, as I always do, because I have caught drug errors on myself in the past. I noticed my Imuran was missing. This made me anxious because I have been taking Imuran since 1988, and now my two yellow, oval fifty-milligram tablets were not in my medicine cup. I asked the nurse if I could look at my MAR (Medication Administration Record). *There must be a reason why my Imuran is missing.* My chart said, "D/C Imuran prior to transplant." I felt reassured knowing that Dr. Lilly had written the note that Imuran was to be stopped but was glad I'd made sure. *Even Santa checks his list twice.*

As I took my meds, I watched the nurse open the heparin injection packaging, along with an alcohol wipe packet. She asked me to pull up my pajama top so she could administer the heparin injection into the subcutaneous tissue of my abdomen. *Whoa, wait a minute, I'm not ever supposed to receive heparin.* I already have difficulty clotting blood, and heparin is a blood thinner. I also didn't see heparin listed on my MAR. The nurse realized that the heparin was intended for another patient. Had I not had my nursing cap on, that serious drug error could have caused injury to myself or surgery to be postponed.

I settled in bed early and caught a glimpse of the same resident doctor in the hallway, fastening his bike helmet to his head. He came over and stood at the foot of my bed. He was smiling when told me, "There is a liver that just became available. It is a blood match for you. Our transplant team is assessing the liver at this time, and you will know by morning if it will be accepted for transplant. It looks good so far, Christine, but we will know for certain in the morning." It was 9:45 p.m. I called Kevin immediately, who called my mom, and so on. But no one wanted to get their hopes up in case it was another false alarm.

The NPO sign went over the head of my bed again. Knowing that I couldn't eat after midnight, I wanted to indulge in junk food. I dug out a couple of toonies from my backpack and strolled to the vending machine in the TV lounge. The food court was closed at this time of night, or I would have indulged in Booster Juice and crispy BBQ chicken wings. Instead, I settled for a bottle of fruit punch and a pouch of peanut M&Ms. I savoured my snacks and then treated myself to a Coffee Crisp as well, knowing I was going to be NPO for a few days post-op because I would be ventilated and unable to tolerate solid foods in the ICU. *I'm glad no one was checking my blood sugar that night.*

After my chocolate fix, I returned to my room and showered. I decided to have a long, hot shower because I knew I would only have bed baths while in the ICU. I even shaved my legs. Kevin has always joked that I only shave my legs when I have a doctor's appointment.

I visited with my roommate, Shelly, and asked her a lot of questions about the ICU, surgery, and the events preceding her kidney transplant. Her calming voice and positive, upbeat attitude soothed my pre-transplant jitters. I tried to sleep that night, but I was an emotional wreck. I wasn't afraid to have surgery. On the contrary, I was excited. I was finally going to be healthy and live a normal life.

All night I paced the hallways on the seventh floor. It was eerily quiet. The hallway lighting had dimmed, and the hallways were barren except for equipment parked outside patients' rooms. As I walked laps, I said many silent prayers in my head to God to *let this be the liver*. I prayed for the family and friends of the person who had just passed away. I was imagining in my mind's eye that the transplant team had a *Human Tissue* cooler with a liver in their possession, just like in *Grey's Anatomy*. Maybe the team was en route to TGH, maybe they were harvesting the organ, or maybe they were here in the hospital, examining the liver. A million thoughts were running through my head.

At 5:30 a.m., I was back in my room, standing by my IV pole and looking out the window, watching a helicopter land, when a young surgical fellow dressed in blue scrubs and a scrub cap walked quietly past my roommate and approached me. *Would today be the day?* Dr. Liau had a huge grin on his face, and I instantly adopted that grin as he said, "Are you ready for your new liver, Christine?" I could have hugged him! We shook hands instead. He told me surgery was scheduled for 8 a.m. but that I should be ready to go to the operating room at 7:30. He briefly examined my liver, heart, and lungs, then told me he was going to autograph my abdomen with a red permanent marker. Now I bore the initials *S.S.L.* After Dr. Liau walked out of the room, the night nurse came in and hung a unit of platelets; it was one of eight units of platelets I would receive that day, to help prevent bleeding complications during surgery.

I phoned my mom and told her the news that I was having surgery in a couple of hours. She also hadn't slept all night and had had a knotted stomach. She said she knew this morning I was going to have my transplant. For her it was mother's intuition. She told me later that, as she was driving down Highway 401, back toward

Toronto and the hospital, she listened to the news on the radio and learned there had been a fatal accident on the eastbound 401 near London, Ontario, the afternoon before. Mom said that had left her with the feeling that surgery was for sure a go this time.

I tried calling Kevin, but my call went straight to voice mail, so I left him a message to let him know I was scheduled to have surgery that morning at 8 a.m. We had previously made a plan that he would not come to the hospital today in the event I was transplanted, because it was Sarah's sixth birthday and we didn't want to spoil her special day. Plus, I wanted to go into surgery with the happy image of my daughter having her birthday party in our backyard, wearing her fancy purple Rapunzel dress, spending the day eating cake and having fun. *Was it coincidental that I was having my transplant today?* I had given birth to a beautiful, healthy daughter six years ago after a difficult pregnancy, and now I was being given the gift of a new life. *Next year I should buy a lottery ticket on July 21, since things are supposed to come in threes.*

Dr. Lilly entered my room while I was packing. He too was smiling. He said to me that it is unusual for a donor liver to be available this quickly after the first liver was not transplantable, but this liver was meant to be, because my kidneys had decided to shut down that morning. My creatinine was 231 (normal is 44 to 97 mcmol/L for women). Yesterday it had been 150. The timing was impeccable because I could have ended up on dialysis. I never wanted to become a dialysis patient, hooked up to a machine that acts like an artificial kidney.

My liver enzymes suggested my liver was also ready to give up that morning (my aspartate aminotransferase [AST] was 958, up from 506; alanine transaminase [ALT] was 907, up from 681; and alkaline phosphatase [ALP] was 358, up from 148). My total bilirubin reached an all-time high of 835. My blood clotting was very poor. My final pre-op MELD was calculated at forty-one. In a matter of two days, my liver function had quickly deteriorated.

The gurney arrived at 7:30 sharp. The nurse assisted me onto the gurney and attached the IV bag with my platelet infusion to the IV pole. I was now on my second unit of platelets. The nurse covered me with a cosy, warm, white flannel blanket just taken out of the blanket warmer. Shelly came out of our room and gave me a comforting hug and wished me well. She too was up most of the night and had a feeling that today was the day. It was a welcome hug because my family was not there to see me off to surgery. The nurses and housekeeping staff waved me off as well. As I gave them a thumbs up goodbye, I could hear my heart pounding as my fight-or-flight response kicked in. It reminded me of how I'd felt every time our rowing crew had lined up at the start, ready to race our way to the finish 2,000 meters away—adrenaline pumping, palms sweating, heart thumping.

There are few moments in life when we are truly alone. The moment before a life-saving surgery must surely be one of them. As I was being wheeled down the hall, past several long corridors, I remember thinking, *This is it; I am not going to be sick anymore.* I envisioned my daughter waking up and tearing open her gifts. She was probably already dressed in her Rapunzel dress, twirling around our house. *I may be missing her sixth birthday today, but my liver transplant will allow me to join her in celebrating her next birthday, and birthdays for many years to come.*

Chapter 12

A VERY SPECIAL DAY

We stopped outside the third-floor operating room and were told to wait. The anesthesiologist needed to see me first. From the corner of my eye, I watched the nurses drape the table and saw Dr. Liau in the back corner of the OR. *A familiar face . . . phew, I must be in the right place.* He was busy preparing my new liver on a stainless steel table. Dr. Liau carefully examined the donor liver. No worrisome abnormalities were noted. *Thanks for taking such good care of our liver, my anonymous donor.*

A nurse put a thin, blue disposable surgical cap over my hair and tucked loose strands underneath. Other nurses were busy getting the OR prepped for the theatrical production, with me playing the starring role, *Mrs. Chopped Liver.* I looked over at the operating table. *This is where I'll be lying soon, exposed for all to see.*

Two doctors appeared at the side of the gurney. They introduced themselves as Dr. Singer and Dr. Grant. Dr. Singer was the head anesthesiologist, and Dr. Grant was the attending transplant surgeon. They shook my hand and commented on the fact that I was smiling and looked happy to be having surgery. Yes, I admitted, I was elated to have surgery. I had suffered most of my life with autoimmune hepatitis and wanted to get on with a life free from my disease and its complications.

Before entering the OR, Dr. Singer talked to me in the hallway and proceeded with the usual pre-op checklist of questions about my medical history, when I last ate, and if I was wearing any jewellery (I wasn't), ending with, "What are you having done today?"

"A liver transplant." I lifted my lovely hospital gown and showed him where Dr. Liau had inscribed his initials over my right upper abdomen.

Dr. Singer confirmed my full name and date of birth, and said I looked younger than my age. *Thanks for the compliment.* I told him I had predicted I would have a liver transplant before I turned forty-years-old. *I was right on the money with that one.*

After our question-and-answer period, I was given the surgical consent form and signed my name on the dotted line. *There's no turning back now.* I climbed off the gurney and walked barefoot on the cool cement floor into the OR. As I walked toward the operating table, I told the surgical team, "Today is extra special because it is my daughter's sixth birthday. I am missing her birthday party, but I have a really good excuse, don't I?" One nurse said that for years to come, my daughter and I will have a special day to celebrate together. *Does the bakery make birthday cakes in the shape of a liver?* I thought.

I clambered onto the operating table, trying to pull myself up while holding my gown closed in back. I started to laugh. What did it matter if my gown came undone now? Then my new liver caught my wandering eyes. Dr. Liau was carrying the liver in a plastic bag on top of crushed ice in a metal basin. He placed the basin on a stainless steel medical cart next to the operating table, in plain view for me to see. Now I was intrigued. I propped myself up to a seated position and peered over to the liver on ice. "Can I see my new liver?" Dr. Liau took the liver out of the bag and set it atop the crushed ice, which allowed me an even better view of my soon-to-be new body part. The surgical team said that patients seldom get to see their donor organ because the donor organ is usually taken into the OR as the patient is being sedated on the operating table. I told the surgical team I am a nurse, and being health care professionals, they totally understood my fascination.

The image of my new liver will be forever etched in my mind. My first thought was that it looked like the liver my mom would buy at the grocery store and make liver and onions with. (For the record, I have never been able to eat liver and onions.) After those first thoughts passed, I really did think my new liver was strangely beautiful. I know *beautiful* might not seem like the best choice to describe a liver, but to me it was beautiful because it wasn't all scarred up like my current liver. I remember making the comment, "It is so healthy looking." I also asked, "Why does it look light pink? I was expecting it to be a little darker in colour." Dr. Liau told me my new liver would assume a reddish-brown colour once blood flow was restored to it.

Once I'd had a good look at my new liver, I lay down on the table and a scrub nurse put two straps across my torso. I felt like I was getting strapped in for a carnival ride. As the anesthesiologist was starting an IV, Dr. Grant commented, "When you wake up in the ICU, I promise you that every opening in your body will have a tube coming out of it." I giggled at that, but knew it was going to be true. I was just glad the lines and catheters would be inserted while I was sedated.

The entire surgical team did a final "time out" safety checklist: Right patient? Right site? Right organ? Dr. Liau verified that the liver was ready for transplant. The safety test was given the thumbs up; surgery was a go!

As Dr. Singer started an IV in my left forearm, a nurse placed a plastic facemask over my nose and mouth. She asked me to take deep breaths in and out. I remember her saying, "You're in good hands, Christine," as she stroked my right arm gently for reassurance. As I took deep breaths and brought oxygen into my lungs, I could feel the coolness of the sedative being pushed through my veins. The last words I remember my nurse saying were, "We will take care of you, Christine, so you can celebrate your daughter's next bir…" Then everything went dark and quiet.

Later, I obtained a copy of my surgical report. I had to know what really went on while I was lying naked on the operating room table, enjoying a very deep sleep—the closest thing to death while still being alive.

With a liver transplant, the diseased liver is removed and replaced by a donor liver in the same anatomical location as the diseased liver—the upper-right portion of the abdomen, beneath the diaphragm and above the stomach. A liver transplant is a very demanding surgery that typically lasts from four to eighteen hours. I was in surgery from 8 a.m. to 2:06 p.m.; six hours and six minutes. It is a complicated surgery because numerous connections have to be made between arteries, veins, and ducts. My report stated the transplant was duct-to-duct, meaning my hepatic ducts were attached to the donor's ducts—like attaching one long plastic straw to another long plastic straw and sewing them together.

Once I was sedated, the surgical team worked in concert to finish preparing me for the transplant. The skin over my abdomen was cleansed with a pink-coloured antiseptic solution to remove organisms. I know I was given a surgical scrub because I woke up in the ICU painted pink. A catheter was inserted, since I wouldn't exactly be able to duck away for a bathroom break.

Dr. Singer inserted a tube through my mouth into my trachea to maintain my airway. Anesthesia disrupts normal breathing, and patients are too sedated to breathe on their own, so a ventilator controls respirations. The breathing tube passes the vocal cords, so when patients wake up after surgery, it is a surprise to them when they are mute. I once had a patient write on a piece of paper in the recovery room after he woke, "Where did my voice go, did they take it out during surgery?"

After numerous tubes and wires invaded my body, the next step was the dreaded incision. The surgeon made a slanting incision just under my ribs on both sides of my abdomen (I have the scar to prove it). The incision is large, measuring two inches to the right and seven inches to the left, and extending two inches straight up over my sternum (breastbone). As Dr. Grieg mentioned during our pre-op meeting in his office, the incision resembles either a peace sign or a Mercedes Benz sign. I like to think that I wear a peace sign over my abdomen.

The liver is located under the right ribs, so my ribs were manipulated as the surgeon gained access to my liver. If I didn't know better, I would have thought the surgeon broke my right ribs, because geez, they hurt during recovery, especially when I took deep breaths. When I was first opened up, over two litres of ascites fluid had to be evacuated from my abdomen. The surgeons prepared the site (with clamps and sponges) and then carefully removed my liver (and gallbladder) from the surrounding tissues and attached blood vessels. *What a big hole this must have left in my body . . . a hollowed-out shell of a person.*

Mom arrived at TGH when I was in surgery, around 10 a.m. While in the waiting area, she watched a doctor unsuccessfully trying to swipe his badge to gain entrance to the operating room. He was carrying a *Human Tissue* designated cooler. Mom heard him urgently say he "has the lungs" and for someone to let him in through the double doors. Four hours into surgery, around noon, a doctor came out of the OR and told Mom everything was going well.

Once my diseased liver was disconnected, it was placed in a basin. *Bye-bye, cirrhotic liver . . . be gone with you!* My body was ready to accept its new pink, plump, healthy liver. The donor liver was positioned into its place. Once the donor liver was connected, the clamps were removed and blood flow to my new liver was established.

My estimated blood loss during surgery was 900 millilitres— close to a litre. Considering the average adult has four to six litres of blood, that was a significant amount. I received four units of type-A-positive blood, sixteen units of fresh frozen plasma, and eight units of platelets. Thank you to all those who donated blood; I wouldn't have made it through surgery without you.

Dr. Liau stapled me back together with forty-seven staples. My listless body was transferred onto an ICU bed, and I was covered with warm blankets. Blood and medications continued to infuse through my three IV pumps and tangled web of tubing.

After the completion of surgery at 2:06 p.m., Dr. Grant approached Mom in the waiting room and said everything went really well and it was a good match. He also added, "It is a biggish liver, but a good liver." Then the surgeon told Mom something that still haunts me to this day. He told her I had had only a few days left to live. Timing was perfect!

Chapter 13

WHERE DO ORGANS COME FROM?

I never gave much thought to organ donation until I was first confronted, at sixteen-years- old, with the organ donor card when
receiving my first driver's licence. I checked the box on my card to
donate all organs. My thinking was, *Why wouldn't I save a life if mine
were taken from me? If I am dead, I can't use my organs, so I might as
well help someone else live.* I told my parents I wanted to be an organ
donor if something tragic should happen to me. I still have this old
paper donor card; I'm not sure why, since it's no longer valid.

Now, the back of my Ontario health card proudly specifies
Donor. Upon returning to Canada, I also chose to once again register my consent to donate because I had been informed that the
progression of my liver disease would ultimately require a life-saving
liver transplant in the future. If I was going to require a new liver
someday, I wanted to opt to pay it forward and potentially save
the lives of others. Like an organ-donation chain! (If your green-
and-white OHIP card does not provide your donor status, you can
register or check your status online at the service Ontario website,
beadonor.ca. For readers not residing in Ontario, you can register
through your provincial, state, or national donor registries.

The Trillium Gift of Life Network (TGLN) is "a non-profit Government agency in Ontario dedicated to raising awareness for organ and tissue donation. TGLN plans, promotes, coordinates and supports organ and tissue donation and transplantation across Ontario." According to the TGLN website, "Though everyone has the potential to be an organ donor, the reality is that the opportunity for donation is rare. Only 2 to 3 percent of hospital deaths occur in circumstances that will actually permit organ donation."

Those "circumstances" typically involve patients who are brain dead. Brain death can be the result of devastating and irreversible brain injuries, such as those caused by trauma, intracranial bleeding, brain tumour, or aneurysm. A near-drowning or suffocation are common causes of brain death in children.

Brain death can be confusing, particularly for families who are confronted with the sudden death of someone they love, because a person who has suffered brain death but is on a ventilator can feel warm to the touch and can look "alive." The heart is still beating, and the ventilator is pushing oxygen and air into the lungs, making the person's chest rise and fall. But the brain has been deprived of blood and oxygen, and brain cells have died. There is no recovery.

I found the concept of brain death difficult to fully understand until I was assigned a clinical rotation in the intensive care unit at Ingham Regional Medical Center in Lansing, Michigan, while training to become a nurse. A patient under my care was on life support after sustaining life-threatening injuries from a motorcycle accident. She was ventilated through her trachea. She had been in a coma for two weeks, and her prognosis was grave.

I was shadowing the ICU nurse the day the neurologists assessed the patient for brain death. Two neurologists had to be present to make the diagnosis. The neurologists performed a battery of tests to determine brain death, including eye movement (none), pupillary response to light in both eyes (none), and pain response to the tip of a scalpel against the soles of the feet (none). They also performed a respiratory drive assessment, which is a measurable test to see how the patient does once the ventilator is turned off. Without ventilator support, the patient's vital signs changed quickly—blood pressure, respiratory rate, oxygen saturation, and heart rate all dropped dangerously low. The nurse turned the ventilator back on after it was determined the patient needed ventilator support.

It was a shocking moment to hear the neurologists declare the patient "clinically brain dead." The nurse maintained the patient on the ventilator and continued with other life-support measures because the patient was a registered donor, and to qualify for organ donation, patients must be on ventilator support to keep vital organs well supplied with oxygen, blood, and nutrients so they remain viable for transplant.

The patient's family made their final decision to donate her organs, as they wanted to honour her wishes to donate. The patient had a red heart sticker on her Michigan driver's licence to indicate she was a registered donor. Every registered donor should inform their next of kin of their decision to donate, because families make the final consent to donate. In most cases, the family will respect their loved one's wish to be a donor if they know that is what their loved one wanted. By registering, patients relieve their family of the burden of making the decision to donate. If the deceased patient does not have family, their donor registration still cannot be used as consent. Someone must absolutely be present for final consent—a family member, friend, executor of an estate, or someone the patient had named a power of attorney.

My nurse preceptor continued to prepare the patient for potential organ donation. She collected blood samples from the patient. To qualify for organ donation, the patient must not have an active infectious disease such as tuberculosis or viral encephalitis. The organs must be viable (organ-specific testing is done prior to retrieval). There must not be any trauma or injury sustained to an organ that will be transplanted.

As upsetting as it was to witness the death of a young forty-something-year-old female with three young children, her organs were able to save the lives of others through her family's final consent to donate. I have spoken with donor families and listened to their stories at organ donation events. Many families have found organ donation comforts them and helps them with their grieving process. A liver recipient I spoke with said it perfectly. "The real heroes are the donor families. I look at it this way: there could have been two tragedies, but my donor family turned their tragedy into a blessing. I'm forever grateful."

While most organ donation involves patients who have died of brain death, obtaining organs after cardiac death is also possible. Patients who meet the criteria for cardiac death are critically ill and are on a ventilator. The patient is kept alive by artificial means, including IV medications and mechanical ventilation. Family may elect to stop all life support because the physician has determined that their loved one will not recover. Or, family may make the decision to stop all life support measures if their loved one has elected to do so via a living will. Once family members have consented to donation, the ventilator is turned off and IV medications and other life-sustaining treatments are terminated. I made it clear to Kevin when we filled out our will that if I were in a situation whereby I was on a ventilator with no hope of recovery, then I wanted him to make the decision to terminate life support and donate my organs.

Family may be present when the ventilator is removed so they can watch their loved one pass. It is important to many family and friends to be with their loved one so he or she doesn't die alone, and so they have a means of closure. Each hospital has a strict policy on the withdrawal of life-support measures. According to the TGLN Act, two physicians are required to be present to confirm death, for donation to occur. There continues to be much debate over the wait time from the determination of death until the harvesting of organs.

Without life support, a patient's vital organs quickly become unsuitable for transplant as they are deprived of circulating blood and, hence, of oxygen, causing the cells to die rapidly. This type of donation does not include the heart because the heart cannot tolerate a lack of blood flow, even during the short time period between cardiac arrest and the procurement surgery.

I want to point out that patient comfort is of utmost concern. The attending physician or anesthesiologist may administer pain medications and sedatives for comfort based on hospital protocol and clinical judgment. The patient is treated with the same standard of care as a patient for whom organ donation is not possible.

Most of the deaths I see as a nurse in the inpatient cardiology unit at St. Mary's Hospital do not result in organ donation; the patients are elderly, have a number of diseases, are not ventilated, and have a DNR (Do Not Resuscitate) order. However, I have also been involved in situations of cardiac arrest that could have resulted in potential organ donation, though patient privacy laws prevent me from learning if specific patients have become organ donors. Hospitals that are designated facilities under the TGLN Act, such as St. Mary's, are responsible for calling and notifying TGLN when a patient has died (regardless of age or cause of death), or prior to death if death is imminent. Notifying TGLN "ensures donation eligibility can be established" and that "[d]onation consent decisions can be assessed . . . before families of eligible patients are approached by TGLN about donation opportunities." In my pre-transplant days, each time I reported a death to TGLN, I would get a lump in my throat and feel nervous because I would think, *Will someone be calling TGLN and initiating the process of organ donation for me someday?*

In most homes, organ donation is not a topic that is routinely discussed—it should be, but isn't. People who aren't affected by it most likely won't discuss it. Organ donation and my new liver are often conversations at our dinner table. My children, as young as they are, have already told me they want me to donate their organs if something tragic should happen to them, God forbid it does. Kyle asked me one day, "Mommy, why wouldn't someone donate their organs? They don't need them when they are dead, do they? If I die someday, can you make sure my organs help other kids?" Little six-year-old Sarah joined in on our conversation and said, "Mommy, I want to give someone my organs too because they help make sick people better." In Ontario, babies and children under sixteen cannot register as organ and tissue donors, so in the event of their untimely death, parents make the decision to donate their organs or tissues. Other provinces and states have different ages for registration.

One father in the Life Donation Awareness Association group I belong to said he sat down with his two daughters and talked about organ donation. His daughters had lost their friend in a tragic horse-riding accident. Their friend's parents were able to donate their daughter's organs, so his girls were familiar with organ donation. His daughter, who was nine-years-old at the time, drew a self-portrait of a young girl with blonde hair and a green organ donor ribbon on her shirt for the cover of a school project. She had decided herself, at nine-years-old, that she wanted to be an organ donor. Tragically, she did become an organ donor at eleven-years-old. She was travelling with her mother, and their car was in a collision with another vehicle, whose driver was impaired. The two were airlifted to hospital in critical condition. The man's wife survived with substantial injuries, but his daughter was not able to recover from her injuries. She spent ten days in the pediatric ICU on life support. She passed away peacefully, surrounded by her family, on Halloween, her favourite holiday.

The death of a child is a parent's worst nightmare. Parents would give anything to have their child back; any parent will tell you this is true. But since all the love and medical advancements in the world couldn't bring his daughter back, this man carried out his daughter's wish to become an organ donor. His daughter's corneas went to two children to give them the gift of sight. Because of his daughter's tall stature, her lungs, liver, pancreas, and both kidneys saved the lives of four adult recipients. She is truly a heroic eleven-year-old to her family and to all the people she has touched. I came across an article on the front page of the Kitchener-Waterloo newspaper, *The Record*, in August 2013. The article featured a picture of the man's wife holding up a pair of their daughter's size eleven canvas shoes signed by her grade six classmates. His wife started the Empty Shoes project to increase awareness of impaired driving.

Everyone is a potential organ and tissue donor. Age, gender, sexual orientation, and health status do not impact one's ability to register as a donor. Even people with pre-existing medical conditions (such as cancer, heart disease, diabetes, and hepatitis) or unhealthy lifestyle choices (such as smoking and drinking) can be organ or tissue donors. Organ donation selection is on a case-by-case basis. A person with hepatitis, for example, may have an inflamed liver and poorly functioning kidneys, but have a heart and lungs suitable for transplant.

I had the common misconception that age was a factor in determining donor eligibility, but the quality of the organ is more important than the age of the donor. In Ontario, as of December 2014, the oldest person to donate an organ is ninety-three-years-old, and the oldest person to donate tissues is 102-years-old! I met a man in his forties at a TGLN summit who had received the lungs of a seventy-nine-year-old man.

Not all deceased persons can donate organs, but many are eligible to become tissue donors. A person can become a tissue donor up to twenty-four hours after death. Tissue donors are often pronounced deceased in their home, at the scene of an accident, or in hospital and are not on a ventilator. Skin, heart valves, bones, and corneas are some of the tissues that can change people's lives. Corneas can restore sight, and tissues can help other patients suffering from burns or bone cancer. The TGLN website states that "an estimated 75 percent of the patients who die in hospitals or at home may be eligible to become tissue donors. One tissue donor can transform the lives of as many as seventy-five people."

One of my patients with a heart transplant passed away after being given the devastating news that he had a tumour in the aortic valve of his heart. He did not qualify for organ donation, but he was able to donate tissues for transplant and the remainder of his body for research. His donated corneas gave the gift of sight to two anonymous recipients. It was kindhearted of his family to make a tissue donation. He was once given the gift of a new heart from a generous donor family. He paid it forward! I asked the transplant team if I am still eligible to be an organ donor and I was told yes, organ recipients may donate.

I am sure you have encountered organ donor posters at a hospital, doctor's office, or pharmacy. The BeADonor poster in Ontario flashes the message that one organ donor can save up to eight lives. What organs can be donated? Heart, liver, pair of kidneys, pair of lungs, small bowel, and pancreas. Some patients require a multi-organ transplant, such as a heart-lung transplant, liver-kidney transplant, or kidney-pancreas transplant, which increases the complexity of finding a donor. The need for donated organs is greater than the availability, so much so that one in three people who need a transplant will die waiting. At any given time, "[o]n average, 1,500 Ontarians are waiting to receive life-saving organ transplants, while thousands of other people await life-enhancing tissue transplants."

At the time of writing, about 26 percent of Ontarians are registered organ donors. If you haven't already registered to become an organ or tissue donor, please take the time to register now. I know it makes you think about death, and about how you aren't going to need your organs when you are dead, but registering doesn't mean you are going to die. Your decision to donate is really about saving lives. I am here today because someone made the choice to donate.

Chapter 14

SHARED BODY PARTS

As you probably already know, not all organs come from deceased donors. There are not enough deceased-donor organs to go around, and without living donors, more recipients would experience further deterioration in their health or die waiting for their life-saving organ. Living donation takes place when a person donates an organ, or a portion of an organ, to a person in need of a life-saving transplant. A living donor is most often a close family member, but can also be a more distant family member, spouse, friend, or Good Samaritan. The procedure allows the donor and recipient to share an organ. *How awesome is that . . . Organs can be shared.*

The organs or portions of organs that can be transplanted from a living donor are a lung lobe, liver lobe, kidney, or pancreas segments (islet cells). The organ most commonly given by a living donor is the kidney. *God certainly had a plan when he made two kidneys.*

Living-donor liver transplantation is possible because, unlike other organs, the liver can regenerate. It takes a few months for the liver to regrow in the both the donor and the recipient. Transplants in adults usually use the entire right lobe from the living donor; in children, a small portion of the left lobe of an adult liver is transplanted. This allows a child to receive a portion of his or her parent's liver.

The better the genetic match, the lower the risk of rejection. There are other advantages to living donation as well. Potential donors can be tested ahead of time to find out if they are compatible with the recipient, and the transplant can be scheduled at a time convenient for both donor and recipient. *How about Monday at ten, does that work for you?*

A friend of mine is a living kidney donor to his twin brother. His brother was diagnosed with degenerative kidney disease. The brothers were considered a good match because they are twins—genetically similar with the same blood type. *That's one advantage to being a twin . . . there are spare parts available.* The transplant was thirteen years ago now, in 2002. The brothers try to go out for dinner around the transplant anniversary. My friend was given a medal from his family that says *Hero Day—Kid Ney and Captain Creatinine.* He doesn't consider himself a hero; he just did what anyone would have done for his or her loved one.

My friend went through the standard process in preparing to donate his kidney: blood tests, urine tests, X-rays, ultrasounds, an angiogram, and interviews. The living-donor work-up is similar to the recipient's work-up. Once all the testing was complete and it was determined that he was a suitable donor, the waiting game began. He had to wait two long years for his brother's kidney function to deteriorate to a certain point before the transplant could take place. My friend was operated on first to make sure he was okay and that the donated kidney was suitable before it was transplanted to his brother. Both twins bear a scar from the life-saving kidney transplant, but their scars are not similar. My friend's scar is along his left side, whereas his brother's scar is down the centre of his abdomen. Scars can be in different locations and different sizes depending on the surgeon's technique and anatomy of the donor and recipient. I'm happy to report that my friend and his twin brother are both doing well. It is amazing what medical advancements allow us to do today—to save a loved one through living donation.

A living donor was originally the best-case scenario for me to find a liver. During my June 25 visit to the pre-transplant clinic, my MELD score was fifteen. I was ill enough to benefit from a liver transplant but not ill enough to be at the top of the list. I wasn't on my deathbed quite yet. Typically, patients with a MELD score as low as mine could wait for several months or even years before receiving a transplant. To speed up the waiting process, and lessen the opportunity for my health to deteriorate, Dr. Renner asked if I could inquire about a living donor, perhaps a family member.

My brother Bill came to mind first as a potential living donor. He is six years younger than I am, is physically fit, has no history of past or present illness, and has the same A-positive blood type and about the same stature (except more muscular) I do. I kept this possibility on the back burner. We had briefly chatted about organ donation in the past, but our conversations were never serious. It was a discussion that needed to be done in person, over a chicken wing supper at Slapshot sports bar.

Bill is difficult to get in touch with. My best course of action is to call my brother Andy. He has a way of finding Bill. Bill knows if Andy calls, it is serious. Andy contacted Bill before I had a chance to sit down and speak with him. Andy said, "Christine needs a liver right now, go get checked out to see if you can give her your liver."

Bill promptly went to his doctor. He later confided in me how distraught and nervous he felt, knowing how sick I was. "My sister was dying, and I was the one who could stop it—the only one who could not only save her life but make her *not sick*. A brand new person as far as I was concerned." While in the waiting room, the receptionist noticed his unease and asked what was going on. He told her, "My sister is sick and needs a liver, so I'm here to see if I can give her mine." The receptionist replied, "I'm pretty sure you have to be deceased to give a liver. You can't just give her yours." Needless to say this conversation did not calm Bill's anxiety.

The doctor gave Bill a lab requisition and told him he should go to the blood clinic around the block and come back in a couple of days. He was directed to the same clinic where I was tortured as a child. Nothing had been said to Bill at this point to distinguish between "donor" and "living donor." I eventually had an opportunity to talk with Bill about living donation and how he would *not* have to die to help make me "not sick." I explained how he would donate a portion of his liver, and that he and I would have surgery at almost the same time. I also explained how the liver is an amazing organ in that it regenerates to almost its full size. I still feel bad about the way he was misinformed about living donation. That would have freaked anyone out.

Bill returned to the doctor a couple of days later, as instructed. The doctor said that if Bill was willing to give me part of his liver, he was going to have to stop drinking. So he did. He told me later, "There was no more pretending that you were going to be okay. You were always sick, Christine, but now it was really serious . . . I stopped drinking immediately." This change meant that, for a while, Bill sacrificed his much-loved social life. When he returned to the pub after several weeks without drinking, it was easy for him to continue to abstain, but "getting back into the social setting was difficult. I was either drinking ginger ale or water, and my friends noticed right off, [so] I just said, 'I'm takin' 'er easy these days.'" Bill also started taking vitamin D and B-12 supplements and milk thistle tablets in addition to his daily multivitamin, developed an interest in chai tea, and paid more attention to his eating habits.

After learning how much effort Bill put forth to adopt a healthy lifestyle just to prepare his body to help save mine, I realized how close we truly are. It takes a special person to be willing to put his or her body through a major operation that would be of no real physical benefit to them. The benefit would be spiritual—he would continue to have a sister who is alive and well. The gift is altruistic. I am humbled and so very thankful I have a brother who is willing to look after his older sister. We may have had our share of disagreements and wrestling matches as kids, but I'm glad to know that as adults, my brother has my back.

My dad considered being a living donor, but his blood type wasn't an exact match and he was sixty-one-years-old at the time. Living donation for a liver is typically an option for healthy people aged sixteen- to sixty-years-old. Older people tend to carry with them additional health risks associated with surgery and post-op recovery. Dad also has a history of active psoriasis. It is likely that he would not have qualified as a living donor. But I know he wanted to help save his daughter and was willing to help in any way he could.

My mom would not have been considered for living donation because of her history of hepatitis A and B. My husband was not a candidate because he needed to take care of our children and help with my recovery after surgery. It was important that at least one parent be well enough to look after our children. Had Kyle and Sarah been sixteen or older, they could have been potential living donors.

My first cousin Catherine lives in Toronto. She is young and healthy, and her stature is similar to mine. She too was willing to be a potential donor. She researched living donation to better inform herself of the process. Catherine is both a registered organ donor and registered with OneMatch for bone marrow donation. When I asked her why she was willing to be my living donor, she said, "I wanted to help you. I figured it grows back, so what is the harm in giving away a part of the liver? There was no reason not to." Catherine only got as far as obtaining a lab requisition and an appointment for blood work. She didn't have time to complete the living-donor screening requirements because my condition deteriorated so quickly—I was scheduled for surgery the morning she was going to the lab.

Finding a deceased donor was a relief. I didn't want my potential living donor experiencing serious complications, or, even worse, not surviving surgery. I don't think I could have lived with myself if I received a life-saving transplant, yet my living donor died or became seriously ill because of me.

Living donation is an incredible expression of altruism and generosity. I am so thankful to my dad, Bill, and Catherine for their selflessness in being willing to be my living donor, but also thankful that none of them had to experience major surgery like I did, or have to bear its scar.

Chapter 15

HOW A DONOR ORGAN
FINDS A NEW HOME

Nothing can prepare a person for dealing with the loss of someone close, and sometimes an unexpected death can be worse. I've witnessed my share of deaths and have observed different rituals and ways in which families and friends say goodbye. Some families join in prayer while holding hands with their loved one. Others snuggle in bed next to their deceased best friend. Sometimes a chaplain is present to provide spiritual support. Death often brings families and friends close in the sharing of tears and heartbreak.

If the family's deceased loved one is a potential candidate for organ or tissue donation, an organ and tissue donation coordinator (through the Trillium Gift of Life Network in Ontario) makes arrangements to speak with the family to discuss donation. The coordinator's job is to inform families about the donation process and to make sure they are comfortable with donation. If their loved one has registered consent to donate organs and/or tissue, the coordinator shares this information with the family. A chaplain, social worker, and family services advisor from TGLN are involved to help support the family in the grieving process.

In the Waterloo-Wellington region, where I live, there is an organ and tissue donation coordinator. At the time of writing, the organ and tissue donation coordinator is RN Judy Wells. Judy explained that timing is very important when speaking with family members about organ donation. The right place and the right time must be taken into consideration. Family members are not approached about donation until after their loved one has been pronounced brain dead, in the case of brain death. In the case of cardiac death, family members are not approached about donation until after a physician has given a poor prognosis of their loved one, and they have decided to end all life-support measures. Timing is everything because families often still have hope and faith that a miracle might happen, and their loved one will wake up and be okay.

A TGLN staff member I spoke with said, "People are comforted by having the opportunity to see something positive come from a tragic situation and often do not hesitate to give consent" when approached about organ and/or tissue donation. This is why I am thankful to my donor family. They went through their own personal tragedy with a loved one and made the courageous and most selfless act to donate their loved one's organs so recipients like myself can live.

During one of my clinic appointments, I read a donor family story that was tacked on the bulletin board outside the twelfth-floor transplant clinic. The article, "Son's choice 'gave me strength,'" was from the Toronto Star newspaper on October 11, 2013. A twenty-year-old University of Ottawa student, Emerson Curran, took a summer job in Yellowknife. He was brutally beaten at a house party. He was taken to a hospital in Edmonton but succumbed to brain death. The family chose to donate his organs. Emerson's father issued this statement: "This is a loss of unimaginable proportions. Emerson was such a thoughtful, intelligent and loving son, brother and friend. Many months ago, in a conversation with his mother, Emerson expressed his philosophy on life and also talked about organ donation. In our immense struggle to make sense of this tragedy, we ask that other sons, daughters and families have a talk about organ donation. We believe that Emerson's end will help sustain the future of many others. His gift is giving us a glimmer of goodness and hope."

Once they have given consent to donate, the family are asked to provide answers to a lengthy medical/social questionnaire about their loved one. The questionnaire is governed by Health Canada and meets CSA (Canadian Standards Association) requirements. It is used to establish that the organs or tissues to be donated are safe to transplant. The questions have to do with any illnesses that the family's loved one might have had and whether he or she was at risk for contracting certain illnesses. For example, did their loved one have a history of intravenous drug use? Did their loved one smoke? Did their loved one travel or live in a foreign country during certain years? Travel history is important because people living in London, England, during certain years may have come in contact with Mad Cow Disease. If a person lived in Africa, where there is a prevalence of AIDS, he or she may have been exposed to the AIDS virus. Certain answers on the questionnaire prompt a red flag, such as having a history of drug abuse.

I've listened to donor families say they were quite overwhelmed with the questions. One donor family member said she felt uncomfortable when she had to answer questions about her dad's sexual history. It can be difficult for family members to provide intimate details about their loved one while still trying to come to terms with that person's recent passing.

After donor information has been obtained, medical staff perform certain tests for disease and disease agents. A blood sample is obtained from the donor to screen for infectious diseases. Certain infections, such as encephalitis or meningitis, prevent organ donation because of the hazard they pose to the recipient. The transmission of infection by a donor can result in not only the loss of the organs or tissues, but also the death of the recipient. Patients are also usually excluded if their death is from unknown causes.

The exact set of laboratory and diagnostic tests used varies from hospital to hospital, but basically every blood test under the sun is ordered on the potential donor. Organ-specific testing is completed while the patient is still vented in the ICU, while other testing occurs in the operating room. Again, each hospital has its own organ-evaluation criteria and parameters.

The organ and tissue transplant coordinator also has the arduous task of locating recipients—this can take hours. When a deceased patient is deemed a medically suitable organ donor, he or she is brought to the operating room. Before undergoing organ procurement surgery, the health care team must manage the donor patient. They may need to administer medications to maintain basic body and organ functions. They keep the donor ventilated to receive oxygen. The health care team also monitors oxygen, heart function, and hormone and electrolyte levels in the blood. Proper management of the organ donor is extremely important to ensure that organs are preserved and protected prior to harvesting, and to optimize the number and quality of organs and tissues available for transplantation.

Transferring an organ from a donor to a recipient requires careful orchestration of several surgical teams. Techniques of multiple organ recovery allow for the removal of the heart, lungs, liver, pancreas, small bowel, and kidneys—usually in that order. After the organs are harvested, tissues may be recovered up to twenty-four hours after death. This process should be executed as quickly as possible because time is of the essence. Commonly, teams are sent from each of the hospitals of the designated recipients, to the location of the donor. Separate teams for heart, lung, and abdominal organs participate. Typically, an organ and tissue donation coordinator, one or two surgeons per organ, and a few surgical fellows travel as a team. The organ and tissue donation coordinator carries with him or her paperwork for organ retrieval and distribution.

Toronto General Hospital sends the organ retrieval team via ambulance for organ(s) in the Greater Toronto Area. If traffic is heavy, which is generally the case in Toronto and on Highway 401, the Ontario Provincial Police will provide an escort. For organ retrieval in more distant locations, such as Sudbury or Montreal, the team flies from Pearson International Airport, Buttonville Municipal Airport, or Toronto Island Airport using the medical transport plane service Ornge. The team usually flies together to the donor's hospital, but the team members do not necessarily fly back together. The team member(s) with the organ return to the recipient's hospital first.

When all teams are in attendance, the organ procurement surgery can begin. The donor is maintained on a ventilator in the operating room to maintain blood supply and oxygen to the organs needed for transplant. Organ and tissue retrieval is performed in the same sterile and careful way as any surgery. Prior to organ removal, each organ is examined for any gross abnormalities that would preclude transplantation. The heart and lungs are removed first because it takes approximately two hours to remove them and they have the shortest viability time, or life span (they are also transported first, for the same reason).

The procurement operation is conducted in defined steps to minimize the cold ischemic time of removed organs. Cold ischemic time is the time from when blood supply to the donor organ is clamped and cut off, to when the clamps are taken off in the recipient and blood flows to the recipient's new organ. Organs can only remain healthy for short periods of time after removal from the donor because cells die quickly without blood, oxygen, and nutrients. If kept chilled with preservation solution (similar to normal saline, but with additional additives), typical storage times are thirty hours or less for a kidney, less than twelve hours for a pancreas or liver, and less than six hours for a heart or lungs. These times vary because of the relative speed at which deterioration begins in organ tissues. It is best if the organs can be transplanted as quickly as possible so organ function does not deteriorate. Typically, the transplant team aims for a three- to four-hour window for heart transplants and an eight- to twelve-hour window for liver transplants. The timelier the transplant, the higher the success rate.

Organs are flushed so there is no blood in the blood vessels, thus reducing the risk of emboli (travelling blood clots) forming. Pulmonary embolus (blood clot in the lungs) is a rare but potentially deadly complication of transplant surgery.

Once all viable organs have been retrieved, the ventilator is removed and all incisions are surgically closed. The organs are packed in an icy slush mixture in sterile coolers labelled *Human Tissue*. The goal is to cool but not freeze the organs, which are then transported to the recipients' hospitals.

Retrieval of donated organs and tissues is carried out with surgical skill, respect, and dignity. Generally, funeral services are not delayed by donation, and donation itself does not prevent an open-casket funeral. No one will know about the deceased person's gift of life unless family tells him or her. Only TGLN staff and transplant team members directly involved with the donor-transplant process are aware of the donor's and recipient's identities. As few people as possible are given details.

Because of the short time available for transplanting the preserved organs, particularly for the heart and lungs, the preparation of the potential recipients and transplant teams also must be coordinated. The recipient's operation often commences prior to the actual arrival of the organ at the recipient's hospital. My heart-transplant friend Andrea was ready in the operating room, lying on the table with IVs started, waiting for the cooler to arrive with her new heart. She was not cut open until after surgeons knew for sure that her new heart was a perfect match. My case was unique in that I was taken to the operating room at the same time my new liver had arrived.

Now that we have organs available, who gets them?

Organ donor registration is stored in the Ministry of Health and Long-Term Care's database and is only disclosed to TGLN at end-of-life. Each province maintains their own donor registration database. TGLN and the provincial resource centre in Toronto are responsible for managing and maintaining the transplant waiting list in Ontario. Each pre-transplant doctor or nurse enters the patient's height and weight, blood type, organ needed, and MELD score (for a liver) into the waiting-list database. Each organ is offered to the highest person on the list (the sickest patient) who matches the donor organ. It still haunts me to think I was on the top of the list for a liver for my A-positive blood type—the sickest liver patient in Ontario at the time of transplant.

Besides the severity of the patient's illness, indicated by his or her position on the list, donor organs are matched with recipients based on certain characteristics. The donor organ should be approximately the same size as the recipient's organ. Had a liver become available from a person who weighed three hundred and thirty-plus pounds, the liver would have been too large to squish into my abdomen. The blood type of the donor and recipient should be an exact match, but certain blood types are compatible. The length of time the patient has been waiting for a transplant, and the distance between the donor's and the recipient's hospitals, also figure into who is the best match for a specific organ.

The recipient's transplant team may choose to decline the organ if they feel that the donor and potential recipient are not a close enough match (for example, the donor is much larger or older than the potential recipient, making the organ a bad fit), or that the organ is unsatisfactory due to poor organ function, viral infection (HIV, hepatitis), or organ damage. Another reason for non-use could be failure to locate the potential recipient. The transplant team might also decline the organ if the potential recipient is too ill to withstand the rigours of surgery. Whatever the reason, if the organ is declined, TGLN will move to the next name on the list.

If no suitable match is found after a local check, a regional check, and then a province-wide search, a search is made to find prospective recipients across Canada and possibly in the United States. Organ and tissue donation coordinator Judy Wells explained to me that TGLN knows which patients are on the waiting list in Ontario, but they do not have an integrated database with other provinces or territories. They also do not have a direct link with the waiting-list database for UNOS (United Network for Organ Sharing), which is the non-profit organization that coordinates organ transplants in the United States.

That said, she does know the high status of patients across Canada. In Canada, the highest priority, 4F, is assigned to patients who are ventilated in the ICU and have only hours to a couple of days left to live. These patients are in desperate need of a life-saving organ transplant and are given priority when organs become available.

If the organ cannot be matched to a 4F patient in Canada, it is offered to UNOS, and vice versa. The brief viability of retrieved organs makes geography a limiting factor, however. If a heart, which has only a six-hour transplant window, becomes available in Vancouver, it's highly unlikely it would successfully make the journey to a recipient in St. John's, Newfoundland. However, TGLN often travels to Ohio, Illinois, and the New England states to retrieve organs.

In most cases, people placed on the transplant waiting list carry a pager with them in case an organ becomes available and they can't be reached at home. On call twenty-four seven, waiting for a new organ. My neighbour Phil got a phone call in the night to alert him that there was a heart available after a one-month wait. My case didn't fit the normal sequence of things. Because I was an inpatient and a doctor told me in person, at my hospital bedside, that a potential donor liver would likely be available for transplant the next morning, I didn't have to make the nerve-racking drive to Toronto for my transplant. I only had to be wheeled to the operating room on the third floor.

Theoretically, eight transplant surgeries can take place simultaneously in eight different hospitals because one organ donor can save up to eight lives (by donating heart, lungs, liver, kidneys, pancreas, and small bowel). One death equals eight lives saved, and over seventy-five more lives enhanced through tissue donation! *A miracle!*

Chapter 16

ICU—HAPPILY HOPPED
UP ON MEDS

At 4:15 p.m. on July 21, the surgical team wheeled me in a hospital bed to the ICU on the tenth floor. I was ventilated, sedated, and attached to a number of IV lines. I had IV bags with medications and blood hanging from poles attached to the bed. I can only imagine what I looked like…unrecognizable. I don't remember much of the immediate post-operative ICU experience, thanks to anesthetics I was given in surgery. When I eventually woke from my surgical trance about an hour after surgery, the first person I saw was my mom. "You're waking up, surgery is finished, and you're all done, Christine," she said. *Surgery is finished? How can that be? I was just in the operating room telling the surgical team it was my daughter's birthday.*

I was scared and didn't know where I was, but I felt Mom next to me, holding my hand. *Mom is beside me… I can't still be in the OR . . . I really did make it through surgery . . . I have someone else's liver inside me . . . I didn't die . . . The new liver works!* I remember these first thoughts. I was in disbelief that the long-awaited life-saving surgery was over, and relieved I had survived.

When I started to come around a little more, I tried to speak to Mom, only no sound came out of my mouth. It was one hell of a scary feeling to realize I had no voice and a tube was blocking my throat and mouth. It felt like the equipment was suffocating me. *A fish-out-of-water kind of feeling!* It made me panic and begin touching the tubing in my mouth. My nurse, who was writing notes at the table outside my room, came in when she saw me fiddling with the tubes. "Christine, don't fight the breathing machine, let it help you breathe. Relax, calm down, slow your breathing." Mom continued to hold my left hand, while my nurse held my right hand—partly to calm me down, and partly to keep me from pulling out the ventilator tube stuck in my throat. My nurse introduced herself as Juliette, in a heavy Caribbean accent. I tried to ask her where she was from, but, of course, no sound came out.

Juliette slowly released my right hand, and what did I do? I pulled on the ventilator tubing again to remove it from my mouth so I could breathe and talk. I was groggy from the anesthesia and was in a post-surgical state of confusion, so I was less than co-operative. I became one of those dreaded patients who pull out tubes, wires, IVs, and other uncomfortable equipment. I detest when my patients pull out their IVs and tubing and I have to reinsert them. Not only does it cause more work for me, it is also uncomfortable for the patient to be poked and prodded again. Juliette picked up a syringe and pushed a sedative into my IV tubing to help me tolerate the ventilator.

I'm not sure how much time passed between my sedative-induced nap and the shift change, but I woke around 7:15 p.m., the time Juliette finished her shift. I watched her give report to my night nurse, who introduced herself as Georgia. Georgia was from Africa and spoke perfect English with a slight accent. She told me the country she emigrated from, but given my mental state at the time, I don't remember which one she said. She chatted with me as she busied herself in my room. I desperately wanted to carry on a conversation with her, but I couldn't, so Mom chatted with her instead.

Georgia said to me, "I will be taking care of you tonight. I have lots of medications to give to you. Are you in any pain? Nod yes or no." I nodded yes. *I was cut open hours ago, of course I have pain.* On a count of three, Georgia and another nurse repositioned me onto my right side in one big, swooping, pushing-and-rolling motion. I was turned every two hours to help with blood flow to my skin and to prevent bedsores.

Once turned, I felt a sharp painful sensation spread over my abdomen. It felt as though my abdomen was being ripped apart where I was stapled together. I needed pain medication . . . something so I wouldn't feel my incision. Georgia sensed my pain and slowly pushed fifty micrograms of fentanyl into my IV. *Ahhh . . . Happy and comfortable again.*

When I woke again from yet another nap, my mom and aunt Wendy were at my bedside. Now I was really confused. *Where did Aunt Wendy come from?* Aunt Wendy said my colour scared her—the colour of a yellow suntan. They let me sleep while they went for supper at the Red Lobster around the corner from TGH. They said they had a toast to my new liver with giant pina coladas.

Aunt Wendy headed home after supper, but Mom returned to my room. When the sedative wore off, I became agitated and uncooperative again. Mom continued to hold my left hand and reminded me to leave my ventilator alone. Georgia came to my bedside, and in her soothing voice, she had me slow down my breathing and work with the ventilator. Being intubated made me panic, which caused me to hyperventilate. Alarm bells would sound when my respiratory rate increased. I kept Georgia busy for most of her shift. I can see why ICU nurses generally have a ratio of one patient to one nurse. Georgia frequented my room, making sure I was behaving myself. Normally I am a calm and accommodating patient, but in the ICU I was not myself. I blame all the sedation and pain meds. Yet, I needed the very meds that were making me misbehave.

At some point in the night, a respiratory therapist (RT) tried weaning me off the ventilator, but, as Mom filled me in later, I would fall asleep and stop breathing, so the ventilator had to be turned on again. At some point I remember motioning for my mom to give me paper and a pen from her purse. I wrote several times that I wanted the ventilator out, but I don't think Georgia could read my scribble. I could barely read what I wrote.

I had a terrible sleep my first post-op night. I spent most of the night dozing off and on. My sleep-wake cycle was way out of synch, not just that night but during my entire hospitalization. Sometime in the wee hours of the morning, when Georgia wasn't watching, I pulled out my nasogastric (NG) tube. The NG tube is a long, clear plastic tube that is taped on the bridge of the nose and inserted through a nostril into the stomach. Having an NG tube made me feel like I had a blocked nostril from a cold. Plus, I could feel and taste the plastic tubing coiled in the back of my throat. Because the NG tube was needed to administer crushed medications, Georgia had to re-insert the tubing. If I'd known how nasty the insertion felt, I wouldn't have yanked out the tube in the first place. My nurse had me assist her with insertion: "Swallow, Christine, keep swallowing." As she was saying "swallow," I was gagging. Afterwards I thought, *If this is what it feels like to have an NG tube inserted, I am sorry for all the times I performed this procedure on patients.*

It was 5 a.m. and I was awake, so Georgia bathed me. She placed a stainless steel bucket of steaming hot water on the bedside table with some white scratchy hospital washcloths, a bar of soap, and scent-free lotion. She told me she wanted to wash me before shift change so I could start my day fresh. I received a bed bath every shift. Fresh and clean I was!

I preferred to wash my own face, arms, and neck—areas I could reach myself without pulling on my incision. The area around my incision had to be washed, but I couldn't muster up the courage to look at it. My nurse had to scrub my lower half because my sausage legs and feet felt so heavy and my incision made it too painful to bend forward. Being on the other side of the bath gave me a whole new perspective on how it feels to have one's privacy invaded. I've given plenty of patients a bed bath, but I had never experienced a bed bath myself until now. Being bathed by a "stranger" certainly made me feel very uncomfortable and timid.

Georgia tried to cover me with a white flannel blanket, but I was too warm and wanted to be left uncovered. I have always been a cold-bodied individual. I wear housecoats and cover myself with layers of blankets in the winter. In the summer, I prefer temperatures above thirty degrees Celsius. So for me to request being left uncovered wearing only a thin hospital gown meant something was different about my new liver. Mom believes my new liver came from a young male or a post-menopausal woman—a warm-bodied donor.

It was 7:15 a.m., morning shift change. The chatter and movement increased in the area outside my room. The yawning night nurses gave report to the awake, clean, coffee-sipping day nurses. After shift change, Mom was allowed back in the ICU. She looked tired. She had spent the night in the ICU waiting room. She'd made herself a "bed" with chairs pushed together and slept with her pillow and blanket from her car. Mom said she had worried all night. She knew the worst of it was over, I survived surgery, but she worried because I was still unstable and looked so sick—jaundiced, weak, frail, and in and out of consciousness.

She sat next to me, and I reached out to hold her hand. Her warmth and presence made me feel secure in the ICU. All the beeping pumps, moaning from patients, overhead hospital announcements, and chitter-chatter of the nurses and doctors are familiar sounds for a nurse. But as a patient, I found the noises bothersome and frightening. It was hard to sleep when the alarms and pumps constantly beeped. At least during the day, these noises were drowned out by hallway commotion.

My day nurse popped her head into my room from around the pastel curtain. It was nurse Juliette again. *A familiar face.* I have a difficult time remembering names, so I associate names with something familiar. I remembered Juliette's name because of Shakespeare's *Romeo and Juliet*. I remembered Georgia's name by singing the song "Georgia on My Mind" to myself.

Juliette asked me how I was doing and if I needed anything. Since I still couldn't speak, I tried to mouth "okay." She took my vitals, performed a head-to-toe assessment, checked my IV bags, and assessed my arterial line and IVs. She emptied the urine bag of a tiny amount of tea-coloured urine. She asked for permission to look at my incision. She was the first person to make that request. My mom veered her head away while I pulled up my gown. I wasn't prepared to look at the incision yet, so I used my gown to shield my eyes. I could feel sharp pinching and soreness across my entire upper abdomen. Juliette lifted the thick white abdominal pad off my incision. "It looks good, Christine." *How can the incision look good? I can only imagine it looks like something out of a horror movie.*

While Juliette charted the values from the monitors behind my bed (blood pressure, heart rate, and respiratory rate, among others), Mom napped in the chair beside me. Mom, like me, can sleep anywhere. While she slept, I tried to distract myself from the ventilator and watched the busy staff in the hallway. This morning I was alert and felt well. My pain level was about three out of ten. I am so thankful to all my nurses for their diligence in keeping me comfortable with around-the-clock pain meds. I can't imagine recovering from such an invasive surgery without narcotics.

While sitting in bed, I heard a voice. The voice was soft yet familiar. It was Nana's voice. All she said was "Christine" then the voice faded. It also felt like there was someone present around me, like angelic hands were gently pushing me into bed. I turned to Mom and tried to say, "Nana is here." I said it a few times, but my mom couldn't understand me with the ventilator in my mouth. Mom handed me the scrap paper and pen off the tray table. I scribbled *Nana is here.* Mom looked stunned, so I wrote what Nana said and pointed to the ceiling, like she was above us looking down. We looked at each other with tears.

Nana had passed away less than two months ago, on June 4. Because she had been more like a second mom to me, her passing was very upsetting. When the two of us were holding hands on one of our last days together, I looked at her hands and whispered to her, "We have the same hands, Nana." My hands had aged from years of prednisone use and resembled Nana's paper-thin, wrinkly, weathered hands. Nana's voice was quiet and she had difficulty speaking, but when I told her I needed a liver transplant, she softly said, "It's a big surgery." They were the last words she ever said to me. It broke my heart to see her dying, but having her know that I inevitably needed a transplant gave me a sense of peace and reassurance that she would be watching over me from heaven. I feel Nana was present in my room in the ICU that Monday morning. She didn't stay long, but she let her presence be known.

Mom and I still had tears in our eyes when the transplant team made rounds around 8:30. Dr. Lilly asked how I was doing, and I wrote on my scrap paper *okay* and *I want to be extubated* (have the breathing tube removed). He told me the RT would be by that morning to remove the breathing tube. I would still have to keep the NG tube in until the next day for my oral meds, but I could have sips of fluids once I was off the ventilator and was breathing well on my own.

Another doctor asked to see my incision. It was Dr. Liau, the surgical fellow who showed me my new liver in the operating room. I barely recognized him without scrubs and a mask. Dr. Liau told me surgery went well and that he'd worked hard to suture and staple me to minimize my incisional scar. I thanked him by giving him the best smile I could muster around the tubing in my mouth. My surgeon, Dr. Grant, also commented, "I told you I would place a tube in every possible bodily opening." I laughed at this comment. It was true.

The transplant team keeps a close eye on their new transplant patients by making frequent visits. We are generally an unstable bunch; post-op complications can arise at any time, and organ rejection can occur while the patient is still in the ICU or years after transplant. ICU nurses are always on alert for any signs of organ rejection in a patient, such as serious coagulopathy (problems with blood clotting), oliguria (no urine output), hypoglycemia (low blood sugar), worsening jaundice, or significant changes in level of consciousness or entering into a coma.

After the transplant team departed, I anxiously waited for the RT to come extubate me. The room didn't have a clock and I didn't have a watch on. *There's no space for a watch on my wrist, it's been over-taken by IVs.* Halfway through the morning, Juliette weaned me off the ventilator. She gradually reduced the amount of assistance the ventilator provided until I was able to breathe by myself. When the ventilator was completely turned off, my oxygen level was 98 to 100 percent on room air. Nurse Juliette was proud of my oxygen satura-tion (the amount of oxygen the blood carries; 95 to 100 percent is normal). She reassured me the RT would be arriving before noon.

I tried to sleep to pass the time, but my back hurt and that made it difficult to nap. I wrote on my scrap paper *Please rub my back and legs*, and handed it to my mom. She did, which lulled me into a short nap. As I awoke, the respiratory therapist appeared. The RT explained how she was going to extubate me. Despite being excited to get the tube out of my mouth and speak again, I was afraid of how it would feel. I had seen endotracheal tubes removed from patients many times, but I'd never asked them how it felt to have a big honking piece of plastic removed from their throat.

Before the procedure, Mom announced she needed an iced cap-puccino from the Tim Hortons and slipped out of my room. *Nice exit strategy, Mom, thanks for leaving me alone to suffer!*

A rigid hollow tube called a yankauer suction tip was passed down my breathing tube to clear secretions that might prevent me from breathing after extubation. This made me repeatedly gag. It was a good thing I had not eaten in over thirty-six hours. The RT was going to suction my mouth, but I grabbed the yankauer tip and did it myself. She knew I was a nurse, so she let me assist in suctioning.

The cuff (balloon) on the breathing tube was deflated. The balloon is what keeps the tube in the throat. When the breathing tube was ready to come out, the RT said, "On a count of three, let's get it out . . . one . . . two . . . three." I closed my eyes on "three," and before I knew it, the tube was out. I tried to speak, but the RT said, "Not yet, you need to have your mouth and throat suctioned again."

The first words out of my mouth were, "I'm thirsty." When I said those words, I hardly recognized my voice. I sounded raspy and high-pitched like a child with laryngitis. The RT told me I would have to wait to drink. *Wait for what . . . ?* Juliette allowed me to have one mint to slowly suck on, to mask the taste of plastic and mucous. It was strange to speak to my nurse. I was able to ask Juliette when I could eat solid food. To my disappointment, I was on a liquid diet until lunch tomorrow. Ice chips, sips of water, and pink, mint-flavoured mouth swabs would have to suffice. I was dying for chicken wings and chocolate.

Mom returned from Tim Hortons shortly after noon, about the same time Kevin arrived.

Kevin was a bit tired from driving when he arrived in Toronto, but he wanted to see me. He went to the tenth floor and asked to be buzzed into the ICU. The ICU is a restricted-access floor, so visitors have to ask for permission to enter. Even when visitors leave the unit for a couple of minutes to go to the bathroom, they need to ask permission to come back in.

Kevin has since shared his experience of first visiting me in the ICU. He said it was scary and overwhelming. There were a lot of people standing around, and he felt very much out of place in his street clothes. The smell, and the sight of all the tubes, wires, and machines, was startling. "I like electronic gadgets as much as the next guy—I just didn't want to see them attached to my wife."

I remember Kevin peering into my room from around the curtain. He looked queasy, pale, and sweaty—his look reminded me of the time he had his blood taken and nearly fainted. He asked to sit down, so Mom steered him toward a chair next to my bed. He only stayed a few minutes, then left. He needed some time to get used to the new environment. *Where did Kevin go? That was a short visit.*

Mom departed shortly after Kevin's arrival. She went back to our house to help look after Kyle and Sarah. The kids were still at our neighbour's. Once Kevin regained his composure, he returned to my room, slid his chair next to my bed, gave me a kiss, and held my hand. Kevin's arrival was timely; I was glad he didn't see me on the ventilator.

It was surreal to have Kevin by my side. Reuniting with my husband reinforced the fact I had survived surgery. One of the first things he did was open his laptop on the tray table so I could read an online news article that he and Mom thought might be a clue to my donor's identity. It was a sad story, but there was no concrete evidence that the person in the story was my donor. All I know is, given the timing of surgery, the donor likely passed away on July 20.

I caught Kevin giving me some strange looks, as I still had the NG tube taped to the bridge of my nose. My nurse announced that the transplant team agreed I could have the NG tube removed. *I already know what to expect, I did a trial removal myself.* The tube was over three and a half feet long. I'm glad Kevin had his back toward me while it was being removed. Some things are better left unseen in a marriage.

Another visitor stopped by in the afternoon. The physical therapist, Gary, brought a walker with him. I thought to myself, *This is much too early to get up and walk. My incision is going to kill me. What if it opens up and my new liver falls out. I'm only held together with staples and sutures.* Thankfully, the walker was for support only. Gary informed me that the task for the day was sitting in a chair and doing chair exercises. My swollen, heavy legs and feet and painful incision made getting myself from point A (my bed) to point B (the chair) an arduous task. Plus, my atrophied arms felt too weak to push myself off the bed, and I needed Gary's help to get to a standing position. But once I had shuffled over to and sat in the chair, it gave my sore back much-needed relief. I suffered back spasms from too much time in bed. I straightened my posture, pushing my shoulders back against the pillow placed in the chair. Kevin rubbed my shoulders and neck to help me deal with the pain.

Gary showed me three seated leg exercises and left instructions to repeat as tolerated. My body was fatigued after one hour of sitting, so Kevin and Juliette assisted me back to bed. Plus, I was in dire need of pain medication. I couldn't believe sitting in a chair required so much effort. One month ago I had completed a sixty-kilometer bike tour in Cambridge, and now I could barely stand and sit.

After a nap, I was looking forward to the supper hour. I had been fasting for over forty-two hours and was desperately craving food. The kitchen staff wheeled in tall metal carts stacked with several levels of supper trays. Because most patients in the ICU are too ill to eat, are on a breathing machine, or have recently been extubated, the supper trays mainly consist of water, juice, tea, and Jello cups. Cherry-flavoured Jello and apple juice never tasted so good!

Now that I was awake and feeling better, my appetite had increased and I was really hungry. It didn't help that I was thinking of all yummy foods I wanted to chow down on. It was late in the evening, sometime around 10 p.m. The kitchen was closed and the pantry was low in stock, so I sent my husband to the nearby twenty-four hour Hasty Market to buy Jello. What a wonderful, caring husband to buy Jello late at night. My throat was still sore, so I slowly and carefully swallowed the delicious, slippery, orange-flavoured spoonfuls. Three containers filled me up. The rest of the Jello was placed in the pantry fridge, labelled with my hospital ID.

Around 11 p.m., Kevin tucked me in and kissed me goodnight, then headed back home. I hated seeing him go after each visit. I so badly wanted to call out, *Please take me with you.* He emailed me later to say he got stuck in traffic in downtown Toronto for two and a half hours. One would expect traffic to be good late at night on a Monday. That's why he left when he did. Just his luck, a Justin Bieber concert had just ended.

Before I fell asleep, my night nurse, Georgia, jotted down my vitals on her clipboard. Thanks to my cardiac-care nurse's training, I knew by glancing at my monitors that all the numbers and colourful waveforms on the screens appeared within normal limits. *Way to go, new liver. You're working well.*

Each shift, my nurse performed a head-to-toe physical assessment. I didn't like being on the other side of the bed, having nurses examine me. I worried they would find something wrong that would mean I would have to stay in the ICU longer. I obtained a copy of my ICU records. This is a typical head-to-toe assessment from my ICU stay:

Peripheral Vascular Exam: Strong and bounding bilateral pedal pulses (4+). *Good circulation in my feet.*

Incision/Dressing: Incision dry, staples all intact. *My incision isn't bursting open.*

Heart: Regular heart rate. *At least I have a good heart.*

Lungs: Bilateral fine crackles and decreased breath sounds. *Those lungs have some work to do.*

Neurological Observation Assessment: Oriented, spontaneous eye opening, and obeys commands. *Yes, I am "with it."*

Oral health assessment: Tongue pink, moist and papillae present. Lips dry/cracked, saliva thick and ropey. Gums pink and firm. *I need some chapstick . . . where did I put it?*

Kidneys: Urine dark tea-coloured with diminished output (total 250 milliliters in twelve hours). *Smarten up, kidneys, and start working.*

Skin: Daily Braden score of fourteen. *No skin breakdown for me.*

My lab results were also closely monitored. Lab draws were taken every six hours from the arterial line in my right wrist. The arterial line allowed my nurses easy access to my blood, thereby reducing the number of needle sticks I had to endure. The less poking and prodding, the better!

All my nurses kept me informed of my lab results, and some nurses printed a copy for me to keep tucked away. My liver enzymes were still elevated while in the ICU because my new liver was not fully functioning yet. My bilirubin was 250 (normal is 0.3 to 1.9 mg/dL), which explained why I was still very jaundiced. My creatinine was in the 240 range, indicating that my kidneys were still not functioning well (normal is 44 to 97 mcmol/L in adult women).

Lines and infusions were routinely checked. I received IV infusions of Humulin R insulin to maintain my blood sugar level, which was elevated from medications and the stress of surgery; potassium chloride, which helped with the wicked charley horses I was experiencing in both calves; dextrose 10 percent in water to provide my nutrient-deprived cells with a source of glucose and water; and normal saline (0.9 percent sodium chloride) for fluid and electrolyte replacement. Nurses repeatedly straightened my lines as they mysteriously tangled themselves into a mess, like Christmas lights.

A twice-daily regimen of the antibiotic cefazolin was administered prophylactically to help prevent the possibility of a bacterial infection. Even with the sterile technique adhered to in the operating room, the length and complexity of the surgery, coupled with my weakened immune system, provided ample opportunity for me to develop a post-operative infection (*which I didn't—I'm glad I escaped this post-transplant complication!*) To prevent my body from rejecting its new liver, I was given IV Solu-Medrol, or liquid prednisone.

Not all of the medications I was prescribed came in IV form. I received the anti-rejection med Myfortic twice a day via my NG tube. After my NG tube was removed, I was given Myfortic crushed and mixed with applesauce in a paper medicine cup. I was on a clear liquid diet, so my Myfortic tablets had to be crushed so I could tolerate swallowing them. To this day, I still can't eat applesauce without associating it with the taste of crushed medications. When I took the Myfortic, I felt my stomach turn. Myfortic smells like skunk and tastes horrible. It was all I could do not to vomit. I tried to chase the crushed Myfortic with sips of water, but I could not get the bitter, metallic, skunky taste out of my mouth.

Juliette knew the taste wasn't agreeing with me as she watched me dry-heave several times. She offered me a cup of rooibos tea with sugar, which helped get rid of the horrid taste. She must have used one of her personal tea bags because rooibos tea isn't a flavour the pantry stocked. I've shared my food with patients. I had a patient crave a banana once. I tried to order a banana from the kitchen, but the kitchen was out of bananas, so I gave him mine out of my lunch. He was so appreciative! I too appreciated the cup of rooibos tea from Juliette.

Prior to my transfer to the step down unit, a nurse from the pain management team connected my IV to a patient-controlled anesthesia (PCA) pump. My nurses had been controlling my pain with IV narcotics, but with the PCA pump, I was put in control of my pain meds at the push of a button. The PCA pump was also programmed to deliver a dose of narcotic at pre-set intervals.

I had another nurse assist in my care my final morning in the ICU on Tuesday, July 23. Nurse Paula was a cardiology nurse who worked in the coronary ICU. She was assigned to the ICU because it was short-staffed that day. During our short time together, Paula and I conversed about cardiology and shared some nursing stories while she changed my central line dressing.

My ICU stay was sixty-seven hours long. Long enough, I must say. During those sixty-seven hours, I was a mixed bag of feelings—scared, tearful, uncomfortable, helpless, and uncertain. The nurses assigned to me were wonderful, and I am grateful to them for their wonderful care and for helping me survive my ICU experience. I hope I never have to experience the ICU again—at least as a patient.

Chapter 17

STEP DOWN—OR A STEP UP?

I was transferred to the step down unit at 11 a.m. on Tuesday, July 23. The step down unit is just down the hall from the ICU on the tenth floor of Toronto General Hospital. I was assigned a corner room. From my bed I had a perfect view down the long corridor. I could watch the hustle and bustle of health care workers, the teary-eyed families, and the patients holding their IV poles as they walked alongside their physical therapists. My neighbour's daughter commented that all this commotion was like watching a real life *Grey's Anatomy*. It reminded me of being at work.

Nurse Sarah was my first step-down nurse. She was a young, compassionate, and competent nurse. Plus, she had an easy name for me to remember because it was my daughter's name! We instantly hit it off. My ICU nurse Paula gave the transfer report to Sarah, filling her in on the details of my ICU stay. *Likely sharing tales of me pulling out the NG tube and confusedly pulling on the ventilator tubing.* I tried to overhear their discussion, but the beeping and alarms from my neighbour's pump drowned out their voices. In step down, one nurse is assigned to care for two patients. Thankfully I was the easy, stable patient, because my roommate kept our nurse fully occupied. He was agitated, liked to yell "nurse" repeatedly, and was experiencing respiratory distress (likely from all his yelling).

Nurse Sarah took my vitals and performed the usual head-to-toe assessment. She looked at my incision while I closed my eyes. "Your incision looks good, Christine." *Every nurse tells me my incision "looks good," maybe it does and I have nothing to fear.* But I still wasn't prepared to see my incision yet. It wasn't really the incision itself that scared me. It was seeing my incision held together by forty-seven staples that freaked me out.

Sarah was called away as my neighbour tried to escape from bed. "Mr. Smithers,[1] you can't keep climbing out of bed, you're going to hurt yourself." "Get me the hell out of this place." "No, sir, you need to climb back in bed." "Get me my cane, I will show this nurse I'm leaving." The patient's agitation escalated as he rattled the side railings of his bed and threw what sounded like a bedpan onto the floor. I was waiting for "code white" (aggressive person) to be called over the hospital intercom. But Mr. Smithers calmed down after our nurse sedated him.

Sarah brought me an incentive spirometer so I could help improve the function of my lungs after surgery. The square clear plastic "toy" has three balls inside, each a different shade of blue to represent the different levels of difficulty. The idea was for me to exhale normally and then place my mouth over the blue accordion tube and inhale slowly to make all three balls rise to the top. I had specific instructions to play this breathing game ten times every hour when awake.

Mom appeared within minutes after my transfer. She brought magazines from Dad and a clean pile of clothes from home. Each time Mom and Kevin visited they took soiled clothes home and brought clean clothes back. They were my laundry service. Mom also brought some pudding and crackers, but I had to hold off

---

1   Name has been changed to protect Mr. Smithers' privacy.

eating until an order was written by the transplant team to change my diet to solids. I was craving food; nurse Sarah agreed that Mom could bring me a Booster Juice from the food court, since I had tolerated my clear liquid breakfast. I had to carefully take small sips because my throat was still sore from the ventilator, but it was so cold, soothing, and tasty.

While I took an afternoon nap, my mom went shopping on Yonge Street. At my request, she bought a journal for me to write in about my transplant and keep track of my recovery. Kevin had put the bug in my ear about journal writing so I could remember the events surrounding my transplant. It was difficult to write at first because my hands were shaky and my fingers were too weak to control the pen. Like my notes to communicate before I was extubated, the pages in the first section of my journal contain lots of scribble. I remember trying to write and having the pen mysteriously drop out of my fingers and fall to the floor numerous times. Each time, I had to wait for someone to enter my room to retrieve it for me. I got a kick out of how each person (usually my nurse or the cleaning staff) would pick up the pen and wash it with a squirt of hand sanitizer.

I woke in time to see Dr. Shah and his entourage of residents walking down the corridor. I was ecstatic to see him. He greeted me with his genuine smile and sturdy handshake. Dr. Shah had last seen me in his office on July 9 when he drained fluid from my abdomen. He and I updated his residents on my health history and explained how quickly I had developed end-stage liver disease. He asked how I was feeling now. "Much better than a few weeks ago." Dr. Shah commented that my sclera (the whites of my eyes) were no longer jaundiced. His brief visit certainly made my day!

The transplant team made rounds mid-afternoon, this time with Dr. Renner. This was our first meeting post-transplant. We had only met once before, at the pre-transplant clinic. He agreed to write an order to change my diet to "as tolerated." He also wrote an order for more physical therapy, to get me up walking.

I had my first post-surgery solid food for supper: a steaming plate of lasagna, a roll, and a fruit cup for dessert. I wanted to chow down on my food, but baby-sized bites were all my throat could handle. It was delicious, and given that it was hospital food, that says a lot about how desperate I was to eat anything with some flavour at this point in my recovery. Ice chips just weren't cutting it anymore.

When my mom prepared to leave that evening, I teared up. She had taken quite a few days off work to stay with me and help look after Kyle and Sarah while Kevin visited, and she needed to head back home to Belleville. Mom and Kevin had arranged a visiting schedule so I wouldn't be left alone. Having someone to talk to had made my stay more tolerable. My nurses were too busy, so I couldn't strike up much of a conversation with them. Sure, we chatted when they were in the middle of drawing blood or changing an IV bag, but they didn't have the time to pull up a chair and have a cup of tea.

The first night in step down was unsettling. The patient behind curtain number two, my agitated neighbour, removed his IV and catheter, and was moaning and yelling most of the night. I felt bad for our nurse, Bricio. He had a steady night caring for this fellow. Also, "code blue" was announced over the hospital intercom during the night, indicating that a patient required emergency resuscitation. The code was two rooms down from mine. I've been involved in my share of codes, which are common when you work in a cardiology unit. I couldn't see what was happening, but I heard nurses and doctors saying things like "epi one milligram IV push stat!" and "all clear." Then the sound of the defibrillator charging and shocking. Nurses rummaging through the crash cart, opening sterile packaging. Doctors yelling med orders. *The sounds of controlled chaos!* Then the sound of success, with staff confirming that "we've got him back."

I also had a terrible sleep my first night in step down because I became disoriented. The curtain around my bed obscured my view and made me feel closed in. I couldn't figure out where the window was, where the hallway was, and where my nurse went when I didn't see him at his desk. I panicked and called out for help. The nurse pulled back the curtain so I could see down the hallway, and left the curtain partially open the rest of the night. He pointed to where the window was—behind my bed, with a view of a tall building with the reflection of the moon on it—and repositioned me with pillows so I was lying partially on my left (more comfortable, partially stapled) side.

I slept for an hour and then woke again because my back pain crept up to a nine out of ten—intolerably excruciating pain. I pushed the pain pump button repeatedly, hoping to give myself added dosages of Dilaudid. The only problem was, the pain pump was set up to administer a maximum of four milligrams of narcotic every four hours. I kept the pump maxed out and now craved more pain medication. *My back is frigging killing me, please make it stop, pain pump.* At some point my back pain must have subsided because I fell asleep again.

The transplant team came to see me at 8:30 the next morning. Dr. Dillon removed the maxi pad covering my incision. Now my stapled incision, which I still hadn't looked at, was open to the air. Dr. Dillon told me the staples would be removed in the clinic in two to three weeks. The transplant team left an order to have my urinary catheter removed. Unfortunately, that meant that now I was going to have to use the commode beside my bed. I was tethered to so many IVs that I couldn't make it to the bathroom in my room without completely tripping over the tubes and wires and strangling myself to death. It was safer to use the commode.

An order was also left to discontinue the patient-controlled anesthesia. Because I was tolerating a solid diet, my pain meds were changed to two to four milligrams of oral Dilaudid every four to six hours. I was sad and felt like I was saying goodbye to an old friend when my pain pump was disconnected by my day nurse Debbie; it had helped make me feel like I hadn't just been cut open.

The arterial line in my right radial artery was also discontinued. Debbie applied pressure for ten minutes because my clotting factors were still abnormal. It felt good to have a free arm, especially my dominant right arm.

Physical therapy with Gary was scheduled for shortly after lunch. Physical therapy was more involved this time around. It wasn't about sitting in a chair doing repetitious leg exercises. I had to independently get myself out of bed and walk. I tried to push myself up and out of bed with my weak arms, but I couldn't muster the strength to do so. My arms resembled Popsicle sticks and my body looked like the Stay Puft Marshmallow Man's. Gary had to assist my swollen legs to the floor while swivelling my upper body forward. I held on to my walker for dear life, tethered to my IV pole. I shuffled from my room to the end of the nurses' station and back twice—maybe fifty metres total but it felt like I walked a mile.

The swelling in my legs and feet and the fluid accumulation in my abdomen had been minimal in the ICU, but for some reason, they were increasing day by day. I noticed my legs and abdomen were expanding in girth. I could push my finger into my legs and leave a large dent. When I moved, even slightly, fluid would splash inside my abdomen. I had to walk with my feet squished into my bright blue crocs, and even they were a tight fit.

Kevin came to eat lunch with me in my room. He brought me another Booster Juice, as lunch was some sort of mystery food. Nurse Debbie came in and gave me a cocktail of meds in a white paper med cup and hung my IV meds. I took so many medications that they were a meal in themselves.

Kevin had taken the computer home, but now he brought it back so I could connect myself to the outside world again. I emailed friends and family, and I added my co-workers to my friends list on Facebook so they could see my recovery updates. I was so pleased to have friends, family, and co-workers post get-well wishes and send prayers. I read their comments several times a day. They cheered me up and made me feel like I had a whole team rooting for me back home. Even friends in the Netherlands and the United States sent happy thoughts and prayers my way.

I was compliant in my physical therapy walking regime. I completed two laps around the unit alongside Kevin. During the walk I peeked into other post-transplant patients' rooms. Most patients were sleeping and connected to a slew of lines and pumps. Lung transplant patients were noticeable because they were the ones with numerous chest tubes and who had the most IV solution bags connected through pumps. Some patients were in isolation—family and nurses donned the yellow gowns, gloves, and masks when present in their rooms. I was surprised how young most of the patients were. Many were my age or younger and looked like they had been to hell and back. I was amazed at how many patients were there recovering from organ transplants. It isn't every day one sees that many organ recipients in one location.

The walking tired me out, so I slept most of the afternoon. I woke when the transplant team arrived again. Dr. Lilly said my kidney function had not returned to normal, but he suspected in due time it would. Dr. Lilly also delivered the good news that I would be transferred back to the seventh floor in the morning—the inpatient transplant unit. That meant I was getting better, but it also meant I would have to become more independent. I was going to miss such personalized care.

Natalie, the night nurse my second—and last—night in step down, spent most of the shift tending to my neighbour. With just a curtain separating my neighbour and me, it wasn't hard to miss what was being said next door. I knew he had had a kidney transplant, and I could tell he was older from his shaky, croaky voice (and from what I guessed were the ages of his wife and children visiting) and that he was experiencing post-operative psychosis: confusion, hallucinations, delirium, agitation. Poor guy! It does happen, unfortunately, and is more common with older patients.

I was so exhausted after my busy day and from the lack of uninterrupted sleep the night before that I actually had a decent night's sleep my second night. I slept until nearly six a.m., when Natalie woke me to draw labs from my central line. It was Thursday, July 25—moving day. After breakfast, my day nurse Debbie helped pack the few belongings I had with me. The porter parked a gurney outside my room and waited for me to search my room for any misplaced belongings. I found my MP3 player under the covers in my bed. I know how easy it is for patients to leave things behind. I once found a bag of soiled underwear and a sealed condom in an elderly patient's nightstand.

Debbie and the porter assisted me onto the gurney, slowly and carefully, while I hugged a pillow to protect my incision. My belongings were tucked snugly around my body, the side rails were raised, and off we went through the maze of corridors and down an elevator to the seventh floor.

Chapter 18

TRANSPLANT UNIT—
CAN I GO HOME YET?

At 12:30 p.m. on Thursday, July 25, I was transferred back to the inpatient transplant unit on the seventh floor, where my journey at TGH began. It was now post-op day four, and I was feeling free. Free from all the machines and gadgets I was once connected to in the intensive care and step down units. I could walk without tangling the IV lines or tripping on my urine bag tubing. I could enjoy some privacy in my own room without feeling like nurses were constantly watching me, even if they were watching me to make sure I was still alive. I knew this was a move in the right direction. The beeping IV pumps, dull scenery, and hospital food were wearing on me. I had been hospitalized for sixteen days at this point. Needless to say I was homesick.

I was assigned to room 120, 7 west, B-side. All the wardrooms and semi-private rooms were occupied, so I lucked out and was given a bright private room with a large bay window overlooking University Avenue. It was a sunny day, and I stood next to the window and basked in the warm glow of the sun. The room was sparkling clean and smelled of bleach. The walls needed painting. They were boring white with peeling paint and black markings. The room was equipped with a large bathroom and private shower. A red emergency cord was strategically placed next to the toilet paper dispenser. When I saw this, I thought of the LifeCall commercial—*help, I've fallen in the toilet and can't get up*. A pale pink-and-blue pull-around curtain encircled my bed. There was a long ledge under the window, where I stacked magazines in one pile and clothes in another. I organized my MP3 player, chapstick, and computer neatly on the tray table. My home away from home, but hopefully not for much longer.

My nurse, Gloria, seemed rushed when she entered my room. She quickly slapped a blood pressure cuff on my arm, shoved a thermometer into my mouth, and measured my vital signs—blood pressure, temperature, heart rate, respiratory rate. She wrote her name and the date on the whiteboard hanging on the wall across from my bed. She darted out of my room when her name was paged over the intercom. Maybe her patient pulled the red bathroom cord?

I was tired of sitting and my back was killing me, so I found a four-wheel walker in the hallway to help me ambulate around the unit. Little did I know, the walker belonged to another patient, and I stole it. *I mean I borrowed it*. The unit was familiar, since I had paced the hallways many times while waiting for a new liver. I knew which pantry had the best food stock. I knew where the TV room was located. I knew what was in the vending machines. While walking back to my room, I saw my first roommate, who had had a heart transplant and then endured a post-op infection, sitting on a bed in a private room. The infection had kept her in hospital longer than anticipated. Her room was two doors down from mine. We gave each other a wave hello and she called out, "Yes, I've permanently moved in."

My walk was brief because my swollen Flintstone feet were causing too much discomfort. When I made it back to my room, I shimmied myself into bed while hugging a pillow to protect my incision. Once I managed to position myself on my back, I used the bedside controls to elevate my feet and legs—only the controls went haywire and I got myself into an inexplicable position, with my head in the trendelenburg position (upside down) and legs up in the air, half-lying on my side and stuck against the railing. It was such a cumbersome position that I couldn't help but laugh at myself. I whispered to myself, *I stuck, I stuck, I stuck.* This is what my son would say as a toddler when he was stuck in his crib or strapped in his car seat. I couldn't reach the call button to call for assistance. Thankfully, housekeeping staff walking by heard my laughter and calls for help and came to the rescue. They too laughed at my predicament and wondered how on earth I got the bed to tilt like that. Bed malfunction perhaps?

After a three-hour nap, I spent the afternoon in a chair next to the window, with my swollen feet elevated on a step stool. It was delightful to see the sunlight and feel the warm glow on my jaundiced skin. My cousin Catherine came to visit around suppertime. She lives and works in Toronto, so it was convenient for her to drive her motorcycle to TGH for a visit. I was desperate to go outside, so Catherine pushed me in a wheelchair to the Elizabeth Street entrance. Catherine had experience steering a wheelchair because she used to work in hospitality at the Trenton hospital—we didn't run into any walls or hit any patients.

It was wonderful to have Catherine's company. We sat at a picnic table in the courtyard and reminisced about Vancouver Island. I hated to go back inside, but an hour sittingand being outside tired me out and I needed to lie back in bed.

Kitchen staff brought me a supper tray shortly after I settled back in bed. I used the bed controls to position myself into a seated position. This time I didn't get stuck. I pulled the tray table closer and lifted the hot steamy lid off the plate. *Is it going to be edible or not?* Nope. It was some bizarre concoction of potatoes, green beans, and mystery meat. Even the dessert wasn't appealing. I think it was cottage cheese and fruit, but I could be wrong.

I kept a snack food supply from Mom and Kevin in a plastic grocery bag on the window ledge—a stash of banana pudding,

Bridge mixture chocolates, digestive cookies, apples, and bananas. Each time Kevin visited, he brought a container of fresh peas and beans from our garden. There were times when the hospital meals were actually tasty, but for those other times when I couldn't stomach the smell and look of the hospital food, I would make myself a whole meal with these snack foods.

Gloria brought me my own walker before ending her shift. The walker was equipped with a seat and brakes, so now I had a portable chair and could stop the walker from running away from me down the hallway. Gloria wrote my name on a piece of white paper and taped it to the walker. *Christine's walker*. She took the marker with her, or I would have written *Do not touch—under video surveillance*.

Not long after supper, my night nurses, Sumaira and Yasmin, greeted me. They measured my vital signs, assessed my incision, and performed a head-to-toe physical assessment—the usual routine, *again*. They checked my blood sugar, and it was a little high, which was not surprising since I had just eaten a handful of Bridge Mixture chocolates. *Note to self: Eat chocolate after my blood sugar is checked . . . I wouldn't want the transplant team to think I am diabetic.*

Yasmin placed a white plastic "hat" (basin) in the toilet and gave me a paper and pen to chart my intake and output (I&O). The hat has black lines inside it, spaced at fifty- milliliter increments, to measure urine. I was to keep track of how much fluid I consumed and excreted. Measuring I&O is one of the tasks we do at work for our fluid-restricted congestive heart failure patients. Now it was my turn to measure my own I&O. I wondered if I was in balance. I had yet to urinate since having the catheter removed.

Just as my nurses had expected, I had my first void and bowel movement prior to bedtime. I'm not one to openly discuss these things, but they are important functions that nurses need to keep track of. No bowel movement in three days could mean constipation, a side effect of narcotics. Foul-smelling urine could mean a urinary tract infection was brewing. I was reluctant to use the toilet for fear that it would be excruciatingly painful. I'm not sure why.

It's not like I had surgery *down there*. But things weren't as bad as I feared. I wrote down the amount of urine in the output column.

There are responsibilities patients must follow prior to discharge. One is watching the post-transplant videos. My room was equipped with a TV, so I positioned it so I could have a movie night in bed. I jotted down in my journal some of the key points from the videos. Yes, I am a keener, but I didn't want to forget important points that could aid in my recovery. The transplant videos discussed physical activity restrictions; walking is a good exercise, but no lifting more than ten pounds for three months. *Good thing my kids are grown and don't need to be carried.* The incidence of rejection is highest in the first three months, and I needed to report any "symptoms," such as fever, right upper quadrant (abdominal) pain, jaundice, loss of appetite, nausea or vomiting, fatigue, increased ascites, dark urine, or pale-coloured stools. Such a long list to remember . . . that's why I wrote things down. All prescription and over-the-counter medications needed to be approved by the transplant doctor. No more dipping into my stash of cough and cold medicines in the cupboard without first asking my doctor.

After my movie night, I tried to settle into sleep, but the incision pain crept up and made me cry and moan. I tend to pant like a dog and make other silly sounds to help release the pain intensity—guess we all have our ways of dealing with aches and pains. My grandma used to spray WD-40 on her joints when they hurt. After I buzzed for my nurse, she promptly brought me my bedtime meds: 1.5 milligrams of my anti-rejection med Prograf, and two milligrams of the narcotic Dilaudid. It was such a small dose of narcotic for incisional pain, but the tiny, round white pill certainly did the trick, and soon I was in a woozy, pain-free haze.

The sound of stomach groans and growls and bowel cramping woke me at 3 a.m. I needed to rush to the bathroom, but that was impossible in my condition. It took a lot of inertia to get this fluid-filled, stapled body to the bathroom. I was just about to sit on the toilet when I realized the urine hat was in the toilet. In the midst of removing the hat, my bowels released. This was the one and only time I pulled the red cord in the bathroom…clean up in room 120.

I always wondered how patients could make such messes on themselves, and now I know how easily such messes can occur. I found it embarrassing and shameful to lose control of my bowels and have a "stranger" see me in such a vulnerable moment. I also felt bad for the nurse who helped me clean up. I apologized over and over. She finally said, "Apology accepted ten apologies ago. I'll make a note on your chart to hold all laxatives and stool softeners."

The pain intensified after the bathroom incident, so I was given another two milligrams of Dilaudid. Around 4 a.m. I fell asleep. I had just dozed off when nurse Yasmin woke me for the 5:30 lab draw from my central line. This was partly why I was tired all the time; nurses kept waking me up at ridiculous hours in the morning. I know they have tasks to complete, but waking patients up is cruel. Yes, I am just as guilty of waking patients up for their early-morning weigh-in or pre-op preparation. I now understand from a patient's perspective why patients nap throughout the day.

Nurse Yasmin drew blood from the central line in my neck while I kept my eyes closed, trying not to let myself fully wake up so I could quickly get back to sleep. I counted thirteen tubes of blood drawn every morning. No wonder we nurses are sometimes referred to as vampires.

The early-morning wake-up call and summer sunrise made it challenging to settle back into a deep sleep, so I went for a walk with my walker around the unit. When I was trekking down one of the hallways outside the med room, I could smell poop. The further I trekked down the hall, the worse the smell became. As I rounded the corner, I found the source of the smell: a big pile of poop in the middle of the hallway. *Hey, just like the dog poop in the middle of the sidewalks in the Netherlands.* I was still groggy and wasn't sure what to make of this situation. I turned around to escape the smell and to alert the nurses to the mess. "It's not from me, by the way," I felt compelled to add.

I continued with my walk and when I saw the tech wheeling the scale around the hallways, I stopped and let her check my daily weight. Each morning I was weighed and wrote my weight in my journal. My weight pre-op was 128 pounds (58.2 kilograms). My weight post-op was 145 pounds (65.5 kilograms). Basically, I gained sixteen pounds of fluid. No wonder I grew Flintstone feet and could feel fluid sloshing in my abdomen. I was discouraged by my weight because I felt fat and had difficulty managing my new girth.

Breakfast arrived at 8:30. It consisted of bran flakes (without milk), tea, Canada Dry ginger ale, orange juice, and stale raisin bread. I asked the kitchen staff serving breakfast for milk. She picked up a typed paper menu on the tray and pointed to the words "fluid- and sodium-restricted diet." I had to chuckle because tea, ginger ale, and orange juice were all fluids, yet I was supposedly on a fluid-restricted diet, and besides, ginger ale for breakfast? That was a first! I took one look at the dried bran flakes and knew they would get stuck in my throat, so I took my walker to the pantry for milk—to no avail. Dried bran flakes it was. Good thing I had orange juice and tea to wash them down.

During my hospital stay, my body was like a science experiment. Each day the transplant team changed my medications around to see what combination worked best. Good thing I'm a nurse because I was able to understand all the possible side effects, drug interactions, and indications for each med. But what about patients who didn't have a medical background? I wondered. Did they know what they were taking, and why? Most patients just take what is given to them in their white paper med cup and don't ask questions. But since drug errors can occur, it is in the best interest of patients to be educated about their medications.

Anyone who has ever been a patient knows that hospitals are not restful places. Patients are encouraged to rest to help them recover, but that usually isn't the case. I tried to nap when I could to make up for all the times my sleep was interrupted. I was exhausted. I felt like I had just come off the night shift. Even toothpicks wouldn't have held my eyes open. I was so tired I spent most of the morning sleeping.

Kevin arrived just as self-medication class, one of the prerequisites to discharge, commenced. Perfect timing! I had called him earlier to arrange for him to accompany me to class. He ate lunch as he listened to the pharmacist educate us about all the medications we would be taking. The group consisted of three kidney transplants, one heart transplant, one kidney-pancreas transplant, and me. Each patient had a support person accompany him or her to help with remembering important information pertaining to the medications. The pharmacist threw in several questions during her class to check how well we understood our meds. She clued in that I am a nurse when I answered her question, "How often will you take Prograf and Myfortic?" by replying, "BID" (twice a day).

Self-medication class taught us patients about each and every one of our post-transplant medications. I could see why it was a mandatory class; these medications are to be taken for the rest of our lives, so our bodies won't reject our new organs. We needed to learn what the medications were used for, how to take them, and possible side effects. Anti-rejection medications are taken to trick the immune system into accepting the transplanted organ and to stop the immune system from attacking the donor organ. In order to accomplish this, the medications lower the body's resistance to infection and certain types of cancer.

Patients are prescribed anti-rejection drugs based on the organ transplanted, their tolerance to the med, side effects, and whether they are experiencing a rejection.

I take little white capsules of the anti-rejection med tacrolimus (Prograf) twice a day, twelve hours apart. Prograf can increase blood glucose and blood pressure, and cause hair loss and hand tremors. The pharmacist asked each patient to write his or her name to assess hand trembling. None noted for me, thankfully. I can still write neatly and legibly. Prograf can also damage the kidneys, so kidney function (creatinine) is closely monitored. This side effect worried me because my kidney function had still not returned to normal. The transplant team adjusted the Prograf dosage based on lab results. I started with 1.5 milligrams of Prograf, and by the time I was discharged, my dosage was five milligrams.

Many meds can change the level of Prograf in the blood. In addition to having to consult with the transplant team before taking any drugs or herbal remedies other than those they prescribed (including meds prescribed by other doctors), we were instructed to avoid grapefruit because it can also increase blood levels of Prograf. I do like grapefruit, but I can live without it. Now if chocolate interfered with Prograf, there would be a serious problem.

I also take the green, skunky-smelling anti-rejection med mycophenolate sodium (Myfortic) twice daily, twelve hours apart. Myfortic can decrease blood cell counts (platelets, white blood cells, and red blood cells). It can also cause undesirable gastrointestinal side effects. Myfortic, like Prograf, has interactions with other medications. Products containing iron (ferrous gluconate or multivitamins plus iron) or magnesium (Maalox or Milk of Magnesia) can decrease the absorption of Myfortic if taken at the same time.

Taking Prograf and Myfortic may raise a transplant patient's chances of getting an infection because they weaken the immune system and increase susceptibility to infections. All immunosuppressed patients should try to avoid close contact with people who have active infections. Proper handwashing is the single most effective way to prevent the spread of many types of infections and illnesses.

We were all given a sample-size bottle of unscented hand sanitizer. The pharmacist recommended we wear a mask while in crowded environments. We should have our own towels, and use Lysol disinfectant wipes to clean kitchen and bathroom countertops, doorknobs, TV remotes, and any other surfaces that are frequently touched. *I will have to be especially diligent in keeping the house disinfected*, I thought, *because my children's hands touch everything and leave dirt and germs behind that could potentially make me ill.* As I sit here writing now, I can see little dirty handprints on walls and windows. *Better break out the wipes.*

The pharmacist also stressed the importance of inspecting our skin for any new moles or skin markings, because our immunosuppressant meds can increase our skin cancer risk. I am a sun lover, so this was one recommendation I'd have to try hard to remember to follow.

I had been on prednisone since I was thirteen-years-old, so this med wasn't new to me. Prednisone is a cortisone-like anti-rejection drug used to prevent rejection of the transplanted organ. It has a slew of nasty side effects, so transplant teams try to wean patients off it. Long-term prednisone use has thinned my bones, and now I have osteopenia. I don't know how I haven't broken a bone yet. I play hockey, and that sport involves some hard falls and hits. I have fallen off my bike. I have fallen skiing. I even fell rollerblading the night before our wedding and bruised my bum something terrible. But no broken bones, just bruises! On higher doses my face tends to be puffy, and I have endured water-retention issues. But overall, I have tolerated prednisone. Prednisone can even alter the appearance of some people. It catabolizes muscle, and many people on long-term use have thin arms and legs. In contrast, fat deposits can form across the trunk and give a "pot-bellied" appearance. Fat also deposits on the upper mid-back area, causing a "buffalo hump." Some people, including myself, develop the classic "moon face." I had a doctor once tell me I have a "Charlie Brown–shaped face."

I was prescribed Nystatin four times a day, after meals and at bedtime. Nystatin is best known as "Swish and Swallow." This med is an antifungal and is used to prevent oral thrush (yeast infections in the mouth). In the weeks and months after an organ transplant, patients receive very high doses of anti-rejection drugs and are particularly vulnerable to thrush. The only time I experienced oral thrush was after antibiotic treatments, when white patches developed on my cheeks and tongue.

Co-trimoxazole (Septra) is prescribed as a prophylactic anti-biotic to prevent or treat pneumocystis pneumonia (PCP). It is a temporary med taken three days a week (for example, Monday, Wednesday, and Friday) for the first year post-transplant because patients are more susceptible to PCP when their immune systems are most suppressed.

Meds, meds, and more meds . . . Patients are also prescribed a proton-pump inhibitor (usually Nexium or pantoprazole) to coun-teract the undesirable stomach and heartburn side effects of the transplant meds. Generally these medications are well tolerated and have minimal side effects.

After attending the self-med class, patients are given a brown paper lunch bag containing bottles of all their meds (except nar-cotics). Patients are also given their own medication administration record (MAR). The self-med program is designed to familiarize patients with their meds and ensure they know how to properly take their meds prior to discharge. After attending the self-med class, patients take their own meds and chart the time of administration on their MAR as their nurse supervises them. Med passes are second nature to me, but I knew I had to conform to the program if I wanted to go home.

Friday, July 26, was moving day again. I was transferred to a corner room at the end of the hall on C wing. I wrote my room number on the whiteboard, along with the new phone number. My theory was, staff moved patients frequently to test their cogni-tion. Can patients remember which room they are in? Staff should provide us with a GPS because all the hallways and rooms look alike.

The only sprinkles of colour on the inpatient transplant unit are the two walls I frequently passed when I went for my walks. One wall displays an array of thank-you cards and pictures of patients smiling and showing their post transplant scars. I was particularly drawn to a picture of two young women wearing sports bras, showing full views of their post-liver-transplant scars. Their smiles show they are proud to be alive and that they aren't afraid to hide their new body image. *I hope I am able to recover like them and smile about my scar someday,* I thought.

The other wall says, "In honour of those who gave the gift of life." I read every touching story and looked into the eyes of the people in the photos, young and old, who lost their lives and became organ donors. It is a sad and heart-clenching wall. Each portrait is followed by a brief story about the donor. There is an inscription on the wall from "The staff of the Multi-Organ Transplant Program" that I read over and over: "This memorial is created in special remembrance of organ donors: without them, life-saving transplantation would not be possible. We extend our deepest appreciation to the families who have been able to share their memories with us; a reminder of the remarkable, selfless act of organ donation, and of the hope it brings to those in need."

I had a lot of time to think while I was hospitalized. I tried not to dwell on the negatives post-transplant, on the possibility of developing cancer, having a rejection, or my autoimmune hepatitis returning. As much as I became discouraged at times, and even became angry with myself for having to get sick in the first place, I tried to stay positive. I prayed to God often and thanked Him for allowing me to live and for surviving this long journey thus so far. *Dear God, I still have a lot of life ahead of me. Please watch over me and help me take care of my new liver, and please bless the donor family and take care of their loved one in heaven.*

The road to recovery was extremely difficult, both physically and psychologically. The worst part of recovery for me was the first time I saw my stapled incision. Despite having been repeatedly told it "looked good," I wondered: what did it really look like? I showered myself for the first time five days after my surgery. I declined my nurse's offer to assist me with my shower—I wanted the privacy and to prove to myself that I could manage a shower on my own.

After undressing, and taking a deep breath, I finally found the courage to look at my incision, the permanent reminder that I had had a liver transplant. It was smaller and less red than I expected, but seeing the number of staples holding me together made me queasy. *Did the surgeon go mad with the staple gun?* After whispering a few choice words under my breath, I started crying. My abdomen was never going to be the same. I tried to convince myself that the incision would look better once the staples were removed, but all I could see at that point was a hacked-up piece of meat.

I sat on the shower chair and sponged around my incision with soap and water, careful not to touch the staples. It felt strange because there were a few areas along my abdomen where I couldn't feel the washcloth. I'd been warned that I might lose some sensation around the incision. It took me over a half an hour to shower because it hurt to move and bend. *I should have asked for pain meds beforehand . . . won't make that mistake next time.*

In the hospital, the days and nights merged together, and sometimes time passed quickly. Before I knew it that night, it was 11 p.m. and Kevin was past the 9 p.m. visiting-hour limit. The nurses didn't seem to mind Kevin staying late because I had a private room with two sets of doors, tucked away in a corner. Most staff didn't even know he was there. Kevin usually stayed late with me and tucked me in for the night. Normally our visits allowed us to get caught up on my health status and on how the kids were enjoying summer holidays. This time, the visit ended with an emotional talk and a box of tissues. I hadn't let my emotions flow post-transplant. I was so elated that I had survived surgery and was given the gift of life that I hadn't stopped to think about missing Kevin and the kids, or to dwell on the fact that I was in recovery and anything could go wrong. But it was that night everything hit me. I missed home. I missed the kids. I felt so sad for the family who lost their loved one. Why did I get to live while another family grieved?

During Kevin's visit, and for the next couple of days, I excessively scratched the palms of my hands. The scratching made me want to scratch more. *Was I allergic to something?* I highly doubted it, since I have no known allergies. I had experienced itchy palms in the past, during my pregnancy with Kyle, when bile salts accumulated in my body. This was something different. I kept a large styrofoam cup of ice chips on the tray table and rubbed the chips on my hands to soothe them. Dr. Dillon prescribed an antihistamine, which helped me sleep because it both relieved the itch and knocked me out. Eventually I realized the source of my discomfort was using an alcohol-based hand sanitizer in the bathroom. It hadn't caused me itching before—maybe the transplant changed my body chemistry? I don't know.

The transplant team checked in to see me each morning. I looked forward to their visits and kept a list of questions in my journal to ask. The team always reviewed my latest lab values. During my stay on the seventh floor, my lab values amazingly trended down, suggesting my new liver was beginning to function. Bilirubin and liver enzymes decreased, so I was starting to appear white again, and not yellow. Even my eyes were whitening. My INR and platelets increased, which meant my blood was beginning to clot normally. I noticed my badly bruised arms, where I was poked with IVs, began to heal. My hemoglobin and creatinine lab values posed problems, however. Neither value wanted to budge. Low hemoglobin made me tired and short of breath. My creatinine values indicated my kidney function had not returned to normal. I was still urinating only small amounts of dark tea-coloured urine. The team assured me both my hemoglobin and creatinine would eventually sort themselves out once my body recovered. I had to trust the experts, but I was still concerned!

During rounds on Saturday, July 27, I asked the transplant team if I could try an infusion of Lasix to help eliminate some of the fluid I had retained from surgery. The team was hesitant in starting a Lasix drip because my kidneys weren't functioning optimally, and they were concerned that Lasix would worsen my kidney function. But they decided to give it a go as a one-time IV dose just to provide me with a little relief.

When the transplant team delivered my lab results the next morning, my creatinine had climbed from 150 to 156. No more

Lasix for me for the time being. The team told me that having swelling is normal after surgery because several litres of fluid and blood are given during surgery. It takes about one to two weeks for the new liver to start working properly in order to help the fluid come off, and they see edema (fluid accumulation in the body) in almost 100 percent of liver transplant patients. The severity of the edema varies, but the majority of us have some extra fluid on board our bodies. Oh, how I wished I could open my abdomen and drain the fluid—*tip me over and pour me out!*

The team also changed my blood sugar checks from four to two times a day—before breakfast and at bedtime. I was happy with this change because the tips of my fingers were sore and full of tiny red pinpricks. My fingertips even hurt when I typed on the computer. The meds I was on can cause hyperglycemia, so it was important to check blood glucose levels. Overall my blood glucose readings were normal (except for those times I ate something sweet before the check). Most nurses let me check my own blood glucose. The anticipation of a quick prick from the lancet made it hard to prick myself, but I wanted to participate in my care.

Because hospital days don't follow the same schedule as real-world days, they can be boring, with a lot of "same old, same old," and a lot of waiting—mostly waiting to become well enough to go home. That said, a surprising development did take place at TGH during my stay: the twenty-seven thousand dollar baby grand piano in the hospital lobby was stolen in broad daylight. Three men walked into the lobby with a dolly, and walked out with the piano. The robbers told staff they were taking the piano for tuning. *Wouldn't tuners come to the piano?* The missing piano was the talk of the hospital. I would often hear staff ask one another if they stole the piano. Police did eventually catch the robbers and returned the piano ten days later.

Aside from the occasional bizarre theft, my typical day in the hospital looked something like this:

5:30 a.m.	Lab draw
6 a.m.	Walk to Starbucks for chai tea
6:30 a.m.	Email friends and make Facebook updates
8 a.m.	Meet my day nurse, get a physical assessment, do a blood sugar check
8:30 a.m.	Breakfast, often followed by a walk
8:45 a.m.	Transplant team rounds and morning meds
9:30 a.m.	Skype/call Kevin to fill him in on the day's lab results, med changes, and other matters discussed with the team
10 a.m.	Freshen up in the bathroom/shower
10:30 a.m.	Walk around the halls
12 p.m.	Noon meds and lunch; sometimes a trip to the food court if lunch was unappealing
1 p.m.	A nap, followed by a walk outside or around the halls
5:30 p.m.	Supper meds and supper; sometimes another trip to the food court
8 p.m.	Meet my night nurse and get another physical assessment

9 p.m.	Blood sugar check number two and night meds
10 p.m.	Get ready for bed and attempt to sleep; listen to my MP3 player in bed or watch a movie
5:30 a.m.	Up and down all night, in pain, ringing for pain meds, unable to sleep, very uncomfortable, often confused

The routine was stirred up when I received a visit or a phone call. The hospital can be a lonely place, and I can see how patients become depressed. It is easy to get sucked into hospital life and want to stay in bed all day and sleep. Visits from family and friends gave me a purpose, a reason to get up and face the day. I loved our chats and it felt comforting to see familiar faces and receive hugs, not to mention it was fantastic that my visitors often took me off the floor and outside to breathe the stinky Toronto air.

Kyle and Sarah visited twice after surgery. It was more difficult for them to visit because hospital policy discouraged young children from visiting patients in the ICU and step down units. Also, the logistics of bringing the kids to Toronto weren't easy to figure out. Visitors, such as Kevin and Mom, stayed most of the day, and there was no way the kids could remain well behaved for more than an hour or two in the hospital. Plus, they were on summer vacation and preferred to enjoy their carefree days with their friends.

The first time the kids came to visit was with my aunt Wendy on Sunday, July 28. I had not seen Kyle and Sarah since the day before surgery, eight days ago. When I first saw them, I knew they were spending a lot of time outdoors. They were very tanned and their hair was bleached blonde. They also looked like they had grown.

Kyle's shirt was partway up his belly, and Sarah's dress was shorter than I remembered.

The kids played shy and were hesitant to hug me. They half-hid behind Aunt Wendy and giggled. Sarah and Kyle had seen me sick all their lives, but they seemed scared to see me in the hospital this time. Kyle later told me why he and Sarah wouldn't hug me at first: "You didn't look like our mommy. You had a hole and tape in your neck, and you were fat." I told the kids that I had a new liver now and I wouldn't have to sleep all afternoon. It saddens me that most afternoons, I had had to put on a movie or allow them to play video games while I slept for two or three hours, but my sick, fatigued body wouldn't let me stay awake.

It was sad to say goodbye to Kyle and Sarah. I was enjoying my break from taking care of them and enjoying not having to listen to them fight, but I was also missing out on spending summer holidays with them. I felt bad I couldn't go to the beach and build sandcastles with Sarah, as she had hoped. Or go on bug hunts with Kyle. I had to stay positive, though, and I reminded myself that thanks to my new liver, I would have plenty of energy to play with my kids when I got home.

On the afternoon of Monday, July 29, care coordinator Mary Anne reviewed my forthcoming discharge with me. *Discharge . . . You're telling me I get to go home soon. When can I pack my bags?* Mary Anne told me that Jill Quance would be my transplant coordinator and that I would continue to be assigned to Dr. Renner as my post-transplant doctor. Clinic visits would be scheduled once a week for the first month and then become less frequent. I would have to have my blood drawn twice a week—once at a local Lifelabs clinic in Kitchener, and once at the post-transplant clinic before my appointment.

The transplant team also spoke to me about caring for myself at home. I had already watched the mandatory discharge videos when I first arrived on the seventh floor. Now I was given a detailed *Post-Liver-Transplant Manual* to help me remember some of the key information regarding discharge. I was told I could not drive for eight weeks. Kevin would have to be my chauffeur. I was to avoid swimming, taking baths, or using a hot tub until my incision healed. Each day, I was to weigh myself, take my temperature, and check my blood sugar. Because my immune system was weak, I was advised to avoid crowds and people with infections. I was also to keep my distance from animals and plants, to limit my exposure to possible infectious fungi and bacteria. *Maybe I should just live in a bubble?*

The post-transplant instructions for home were overwhelming. I had been hoping that once I left the hospital, I could carry on with life the way I did before I became so sick—guess I was going to have to watch how much I lifted, and stay away from my pet rabbits. I was looking forward to gardening though. I was sure my flower gardens were in desperate need of deadheading and weeding. I would just have to don a mask and gloves first.

Some patients require additional physical therapy and recovery time and go to a rehabilitation hospital after they are discharged, but most are able to go directly home from the hospital. I was one of the latter. A physical therapist assessed my mobility and ability to return home safely. She had me walk up and down stairs in the stairwell because we have a three-storey house. I was a little nervous about navigating the concrete stairs—it was a long way down to the lower level. The physical therapist showed me how to walk sideways up and down the stairs by facing the railing and placing one foot at a time on each step. I was slow-moving but passed the stair assessment with flying colours.

I also purposely went for walks in the hallways when I knew the transplant team was rounding on other patients. I would casually strut my stuff and walk by the transplant team, showing off to them. It was my way of indicating to the team that *Hey, I can walk on my own, no problems—please let me go home soon.* They noticed! One doctor commented that I was walking well and he was glad to see me up and about.

On the night of July 29, or sometime in the wee hours of July 30, I got very confused and disoriented after a bizarre dream. I dreamt that all the fluid in my body gushed out and covered my room in water, like a water main break. The cleaning staff had to mop up the fluid and put a yellow *Caution* sign at my doorway. I woke up and realized that I hadn't burst open and was still swollen with fluids. I remembered dreaming that I was going to get in trouble because I didn't properly keep track of my fluids in the output section of my chart. I panicked and pushed the call button for my nurse, who turned on the lights, helped calm me down, and used pillows to reposition me in bed. She also gave me some pain medication because I was now hurting from flailing in bed during my dream.

On Tuesday, July 30, while I was eating breakfast, a surprise visitor popped in: my old roommate Shelly was at TGH for her first post-op clinic appointment. I was feeling pretty miserable that morning after a bad night's sleep, but Shelly's cheerful smile and big hugs brightened my day. Shelly provided me with an update on her progress. Seeing her doing so well post-op was encouraging.

The transplant team made their usual morning rounds, and this time they discussed the possibility of my being discharged on Friday—only three days away! The only thing interfering with discharge was my high creatinine levels. *Okay, kidneys, did you hear that? Smarten up and start working.*

I informed Dr. Lilly of my weird dreams, drowsiness, and lack of sleep, and the fact that Dilaudid was making me dazed and confused after taking it. Dr. Lilly suggested changing my pain meds to the narcotic Percocet, a combination of oxycodone and acetaminophen. Percocet ended up being my drug of choice for controlling incision pain and back pain. I felt more alert and wasn't so drowsy after taking it. Bizarre dreams and confusion still occurred in the night, but they were likely a function of being in the hospital's unfamiliar and disruptive sleeping environment.

The next day, Wednesday, July 31, Dr. Lilly asked if I would be willing to volunteer to allow one of his medical students to practise his health-history and physical examination skills on a live patient. I thought being a guinea pig would be fun and was honoured that Dr. Lilly thought I would make a good patient to practise on. Dr. Lilly sat on a chair in the corner of my room and took notes. The medical student asked a long, detailed list of questions pertaining to my past illnesses, current complaints, surgical history, and so forth. I sometimes went off on a tangent and offered too much information. I was using too much medical jargon when I was supposed to pretend I was the common patient. The medical student jokingly commented that I was making this too easy for him.

The medical student also demonstrated his physical-assessment skills to Dr. Lilly. He performed a comprehensive head-to-toe physical exam, using my body as the model. I tried to keep quiet and not giggle when he poked a tickly spot. After the assessment, Dr. Lilly taught his student how to assess for ascites, and how to palpate my new liver. I didn't like my new liver being touched; it was still so foreign to me that, even though I knew it didn't make sense to feel this way, I was afraid it would become detached from my body.

Dr. Lilly and his medical student had a few minutes to spare and were able to stay in my room and chat. I so enjoyed having their undivided attention and was able to ask them a couple of strange questions. Primarily, I wanted to know whether I still had autoimmune hepatitis. Dr. Lilly explained to me that technically, I no longer had autoimmune hepatitis, but there was always a possibility the disease could return. *What . . . I don't have a liver disease anymore . . . I don't remember life without liver disease, and now you're telling me it's gone . . . how cool is that?* The thing is, if my disease did return, the doctors wouldn't be able to easily distinguish between the return of my disease and a rejection of my new liver. Both complications cause the same symptoms, including jaundice, elevated liver enzymes, ascites, fatigue, and right upper abdominal pain. However, if I ever do experience the return of my disease or a rejection, the treatment is the same—an increase in my anti-rejection meds.

Mom, Grandma, Kyle, and Sarah came to visit in the late afternoon and through the supper hour. Grandma brought a quart of delicious fresh raspberries picked from her garden—my all-time favourite food. I had to wait and indulge in my berries after my evening blood sugar was checked. The kids were wildly boisterous, so we took them to the food court to run off some steam. It was raining, or we would have sent them outside to run around. They had pent-up energy from their two-hour car trip. My kids have a thing for walkers, I don't know why. Whenever they have access to a walker, they feel they need to use it as a go-cart. One kid would sit on my walker while the other pushed, often into walls. *Crash up derby, hospital style.* Good thing my secluded corner room was at the end of the unit and tucked away behind two doors, so we didn't disturb other patients. When they left, I walked them to the elevator. Mom laughed at Grandma and me as we slowly walked, side by side, pushing our walkers. Like Grandma, like granddaughter. As we made our way down the hall, we saw Natalie (my nurse from the step down unit), at the nurses' station. I introduced her to Kyle and Sarah. She knelt down next to Sarah and took her tiny hand and said, "You take good care of your mommy for me." Sarah gave a shy grin and nodded When I hugged the kids goodbye, Sarah said, "Mommy, you have a nice nurse." *Yes I do, Sarah.*

At this point in my recovery, I still had one dreadfully annoying piece of plastic tubing to deal with—the central line. The transplant team was waiting for my platelets and INR to increase before allowing the central line to be removed so my blood would clot after its removal. I asked if I could remove it, just to see their response. Dr. Lilly said with a chuckle, "Remember, you're the patient."

Student nurse Caitlin, under supervision of a more senior nurse, was given the thumbs-up to remove the central line. I've removed central lines many times and was dreading this procedure, even though patients seem to tolerate the procedure fairly well and have reported that the peeling of the tape off their skin and the removal of the sutures in their neck were worse than pulling out the long tube.

Those patients' reports were right. The worst was getting the dressing out of my hair. Caitlin had to give my hair a little trim. There was a lot of tugging and snipping as she removed the five black sutures sewn into my skin that were holding the tubing against the right side of my neck. After she slid the long, white, hollow catheter tube out of my internal jugular vein in one long pull, covered the site with a large square of white gauze, and began maintaining manual pressure on it, her name and the supervising nurse's name were paged over the intercom. One of their patients was yelling for help because she was short of breath and having chest pain. Caitlin said to me, "You're a nurse, I trust you to keep pressure on the site." I took over the task as she darted out of my room. I had to lie flat for thirty minutes to reduce my risk of developing a potentially fatal air embolism (air in a blood vessel).

Although the transplant team had figured my discharge date would be Friday, August 2, twelve days post-op, during rounds on Thursday they agreed that there was no reason to keep me another day since my creatinine, although still not normal, was trending downward. My response: "What time can I leave?" After twenty-two days in the hospital, I was ready to get this ball rolling.

There were a few items to wrap up before discharge. First, I needed a ride. I was immediately on the phone with Kevin. It was a good driving day on Highway 401, and he arrived in less than two hours. While waiting for Kevin, I packed. Kevin arrived mid-morning and hurriedly packed the rest of my bags and took them out to the car. He wanted to leave Toronto promptly while the driving was good. However, there were a couple of holdups.

First, I had to wait for my morning Prograf level result in case the transplant team needed to change the dose. My Prograf level was within normal limits, so no changes were made.

Second, I had to review meds with the transplant pharmacist. The pharmacist, David, watched me open the brown paper bag full of meds. I dumped out the bottles and blister packs onto the tray table and lined them up alongside the MAR sheet he provided. One by one, I told David the name of each drug, its use, when to take it, and possible side effects. Based on the speed and thoroughness of my review, he said, "You must be a nurse or work in health care, Christine." "A nurse." "That explains why you know your meds so well." Plus, I wanted to leave ASAP and knew a good review performance would speed things along. I have to say, the self-administration program is a great way to promote patient independence, ensure patients know their medications, and help them feel comfortable taking their meds, which is important because they will be taking them for life.

Nurse Cathy freed me from the last IV that occupied my body. It felt weird to have nothing attached to my arms, but good to finally be free of all tethers. I underwent MRSA screening (my nose, armpits, and bottom were swabbed), which checks for an antibiotic-resistant bacterium that is especially troublesome in hospitals. It can take root in patients who have weakened immune systems. I never learned the results, so I assume I am not a MRSA carrier, phew!

Meanwhile, Kevin was searching the halls for a wheelchair, which is like digging for gold. It was a long walk to the car and I wasn't confident I would make it. Kevin told me to take my time and offered his arm for support. As we passed the nurses' station, I waved goodbye. *Yeah, I'm outta here!* On our way to the elevator I spotted a vacant wheelchair sitting in the main hallway. *This can't be, no one is around and there is a wheelchair . . . It must be waiting for me.* I planted myself in the wheelchair and told Kevin to make a run for it—to our getaway car!

He parked me outside at the Elizabeth Street pickup and drop-off point while he fetched our car. Kevin assisted me into the car, and we left the wheelchair outside for someone else to stumble upon. The water baby I was still carrying in my abdomen required me to angle the passenger seat slightly back. Kevin placed pillows behind my back and under my feet. I took a Percocet to help ease the discomfort I knew the drive would cause. It was 1 p.m. We thought we were leaving in good time to miss rush hour, but it should just be assumed that Highway 401 is always a huge parking lot—the trip home took over three hours. Thankfully I slept most of the way.

Chapter 19

THERE'S NO PLACE LIKE HOME

Returning home after twenty-two days in hospital was a strange mix of comfort and difficulty. When I entered our house for the first time, I walked around the main floor and touched the basil-coloured walls and antique furniture. I picked up a couple of knick-knacks we had acquired from family vacations abroad. I needed to reassure myself that I was actually home. Everything seemed surreal. I was taken aback by the smell and colour—my senses were working overtime because the hospital had dulled them with its pastel-coloured walls and pungent smells. Seeing vibrant colours again, and smelling the sweetness of freshly cut grass, blowing through the open windows, was powerful.

I opened our sliding glass door in the kitchen and stepped outside into our backyard. Kevin helped me down the steps, and I used the wooden potting bench near the door for support. I had night-mares of falling and opening up my incision, so I took it easy. The songbirds happily tweeted as if they were welcoming me home. A couple of grey squirrels played tag as they chased each other around the catalpa tree. I stood on our patio and took some deep breaths of fresh air. *I missed this outdoor smell.* I cautiously walked around our yard and looked at the flowerbeds. I tried not to focus on the dandelions that had intruded the flowerbeds, or the fact that many flowers did, as I'd suspected, need deadheading. I stood looking at my crazy daisies, with tears running down my cheeks, thinking, *Without my new liver, I wouldn't be here on this warm summer's day, enjoying my flowers. Thank you, donor family.*

My legs were still weak and my gait unsteady and stiff. I wandered slowly over to the bunny huts to visit my pet rabbits Snowy, Tigger, and Eeyore. They are outdoor lionhead lop bunnies and live in cedar rabbit huts. I apologized to the bunnies for their having to be cooped up. I usually let them run free around our large fenced yard for exercise and weed control. I knew they wouldn't be allowed out of their huts anytime soon. I was in no shape to chase them out of our gardens or corral them back into their huts. I was told immediately post-transplant that I wasn't supposed to pick up and snuggle with my bunnies in case I acquired some sort of infection from them, but I couldn't help but pet my cute furry pets. I had missed them. They'd missed me too, and soaked up all the petting and nose-rubbing. I made sure I washed my hands with soap and water afterwards, and gave my hands a few extra squirts of hand sanitizer, just in case.

Kyle and Sarah weren't home. We had sent them to my parents' house in Belleville. My family knew I would need quiet and relaxation my first weeks at home. I missed them and wanted nothing more than to be wrapped in their little arms, but I was too weak and tired for their level of energy and enthusiasm just yet. Those first few weeks at home, I slept at least ten hours every night, and had a nap in the morning and a longer nap in the afternoon. Part of the reason I slept so much was that Percocet made me sleepy. I tried to reduce the number of Percocet tablets I took each day, but without pain medication, I was miserable. Having forty-seven staples embedded in my skin and having an incision the width of my abdomen warranted opiates.

One of the post-transplant requirements was to check my blood sugar twice a day, just as the nurses and I had done in the hospital.

I still really hated poking my fingertips before breakfast and in the evening to obtain a blood sample, but I knew I was susceptible to developing diabetes because of my high dosages of prednisone and Prograf and because I had a history of gestational diabetes. My sugars were well controlled. I did make a conscious effort to limit the amount of carbohydrates I consumed and to drink water instead of chocolate milk and juice. Not only was I watching my sugar intake, but I was also once again on a sodium-restricted diet because of fluid-retention issues. So I couldn't eat sugar or salt. *Might as well eat cardboard.* I ate mostly vegetables from our garden, and meat— plain garden salads, plain chicken, plain hamburger.

My taste buds changed after surgery. Foods I had detested, I now enjoyed eating. Maybe my donor liked vegetables and I acquired his or her fondness for salad. I loved salad and couldn't get enough of it. I also craved potato chips. I was never a big potato-chip eater, but now I craved the crispy saltiness. I would allow myself only a handful of salt-and-vinegar or low-salt chips—enough to satisfy my craving but not enough to ruin my low-sodium diet.

It wasn't just new cravings that were peculiar. I also tasted soap and metal. If I used a fork or spoon, I tasted metal. If I touched a tin can, I tasted metal. If I washed my hands with soap, I tasted it. I love Bath & Body Works scented soaps, especially Coconut Cove and Berry Sangria. But when I washed my hands with them, coconut or berry soapy tastes lingered in my mouth. It was horrible washing the dishes; I could taste the metal utensils and pots along with the dish detergent. It was a rather odd phenomenon. *Were my meds causing this? Were my electrolytes out of balance? Was there something wrong with my salivary glands?* Like many patients, I resorted to Google to try and diagnose myself. This symptom wasn't something I had encountered in my nursing practice. I tried to google *strange soapy metallic taste* but didn't find any concrete medical explanation, only a bunch of blogs from people who had experienced the same phenomenon. *Good, I'm not the only crazy person with this problem.* But then the soapy and metallic tastes disappeared after about a month, and I could use my favourite soaps and utensils again without tasting them.

It's funny the things you take for granted during recovery after a major surgery. In the hospital, I had had the luxury of having a raised toilet with handrails on the wall. The first few times I sat on our toilet at home, I had to practically fall backwards onto it since it was significantly lower and my legs were too weak to support my body into a sitting position. *Was our toilet always this low?* Without handrails, I had to improvise and used the sink vanity for support. I was afraid I was going to rip the vanity off the wall. I was also afraid of dislocating my atrophied shoulders when I pulled myself up. *Maybe I should rent a toilet seat riser . . . No, that's for an old person.*

My first day at home was tiresome, as I endured more activity than I had in a long time. That night I was so looking forward to sleeping in my pillowtop bed and snuggling under my fresh bed-sheets. As I shimmied my way into bed, I went to reach for the side railing to assist myself. *Oh right, I'm not in a hospital bed.* Kevin helped me position myself so I was lying on my left side with a pillow under my fluid-filled abdomen, a pillow between my swollen knees, a pillow along my back, and two pillows under my head and bony shoulders. With so many pillows, there was no room for Kevin beside me. Poor Kevin, my wonderful husband and caretaker, had to sleep downstairs on our lumpy futon for a month.

I quickly drifted off to sleep, but woke two hours later to use the bathroom. There was one problem, however. I couldn't get out of bed. *I stuck, I stuck, I stuck again.* I was used to using the bed controls and side railings to prop myself into a seated position. I didn't have the strength to assist my swollen and sore body upright. I had to yell for Kevin to come help. He wasn't happy that I called him away from his BC Lions football game. Kevin assisted me to the bathroom and then rearranged my pillow tower so I could go back to sleep.

I woke several times—to get comfortable, to take Percocet, to use the bathroom. Around 5:30 a.m., when the sun was starting to peek out, I woke in a panic. I was disoriented, alone, and afraid. In my half-asleep, Percocet-induced haze, I still thought I was in the hospital. *Where am I? Why didn't my nurse come check on me? Why is no one coming to give me Percocet?* My body was sopping wet with sweat and I was trembling. *What if something bad happens? I don't have a call button. What if my new liver stops working, what do I do? What if my incision bursts open and I bleed to death, who do I call?* I was so frightened that I literally jumped out of bed, and injured my left shoulder in doing so. I walked to the window and opened the blinds. The darkness was freaking me out. I needed to see outside. It wasn't the bustling University Avenue out there—taxis honking at each other, pedestrians hurrying to work, homeless people rummaging in garbage cans. It was our quiet crescent, lined with single-family detached homes, and a grassy area in the middle of our cul-de-sac with a streetlight and a maple tree. Yes, I was home.

Every morning I weighed myself on the digital glass bathroom scale. My morning weigh-ins reminded me of my rowing days, when we crew members had to weigh ourselves to make sure we maintained our lightweight status of 125 pounds or under. Day one, I reluctantly stepped onto the scale and looked over the top of my swollen belly to see my weight light up in bright red: 145.8 pounds. *What the . . .* I was 128 pounds before surgery. I told myself, *I'm still my slim self underneath all this fluid.* I couldn't take Lasix to help eliminate the excess fluid because I was still having issues with my kidney function. I waddled downstairs and took my temperature: 36.6 degrees Celsius, no fever. Then I poked myself: blood sugar 5.6, well controlled. Every morning I was to follow this routine of monitoring myself. Rejection, return of my disease, infection, and complications are possible anytime post-transplant, so it was, and will forever be, imperative to keep a close eye on myself and report any problems to my transplant coordinator via Easy Call.

Easy Call is my lifeline to my transplant team. I dial a 416 Toronto phone number, enter my PIN and password, and voila, with a few prompts, I can leave a message for my transplant coordinator, Registered Nurse Jill Quance. Easy Call is the Multi-Organ Transplant Program's patient communication system. I like to think of it as my tele-nurse. I call Jill with concerns or questions, and Jill calls me with medication changes, appointments, and lab results. During my first week at home, Jill called almost daily to inform me of changes in my medications and dosages. If I wasn't home, or was sleeping and turned the ringer off, and she left a voice-mail message instead of speaking to me directly, Easy Call would call every hour until I answered. After I listened to the message, I had to repeat it so Jill would know I got the message and understood it.

My initial medication combination didn't agree with me—my hemoglobin and white blood cell count remained low, and my kidney function failed to improve. There were many medication changes those first months post-transplant. Good thing I'm a nurse and I am used to keeping track of medications, or I would have had difficulty managing my twenty-five pills a day. I tried keeping them in a plastic weekly pill organizer, but I had so many medication changes that I found I had to re-sort the pill compartments often. Instead, I organized all my pill bottles and packages into a colourful wicker basket on top of the fridge so they were accessible for my morning and evening med passes. I know my kids had access to my medications, but I sat down with them and talked to them about my meds and explained that my meds make me better, but would make them sick. Kevin tried to frighten the kids and told them if they took my meds they would have to go to the hospital and have their right arm cut off. I'd be scared too if I were told that.

I *grudgingly* had labs drawn three times a week, on Mondays, Wednesdays, and Fridays. Jill left frequent messages to inform me of my lab results as well as medication changes. Those darn old kidneys were stubborn and didn't want to work properly. My creatinine wouldn't budge for weeks. I needed my creatinine to be under ninety-seven for it to be normal, and it was around 160. My kidneys really did take a pounding pre-transplant. My poor kidney function caused anemia (low hemoglobin). Hemoglobin for a normal, healthy female should be over 123 g/L. Now my hemoglobin was in the seventies. No wonder I was tired, pale, and really short of breath when I walked up stairs.

My Prograf level had to be checked often to ensure I was receiving a therapeutic dose. My liver enzymes were monitored for rejection or return of my autoimmune hepatitis. My hemoglobin, white blood cell count, INR, platelets, electrolytes, and so on were all monitored. My numbers were by no means within normal limits at first because my new liver wasn't working optimally yet. Dr. Lilly told me it would take at least two weeks for my new liver to start to work. My new liver had to adjust to its new home, and my body had to be willing to accept its new body part.

On Friday, August 9, only nine days out of hospital, I returned to St. Mary's ER because my hemoglobin dipped to sixty-two—dangerously low. My co-worker, and friend, Melyssa drove me to the ER because Kevin was at work. I tried to imagine she was giving me a lift to work and not to the hospital as a patient. Dr. Renner faxed orders to transfuse three units of packed red blood cells, with twenty milligrams of IV Lasix between the first and second units and after the third unit. I had massive ascites, and the Lasix between the blood units helped prevent my body from retaining additional fluid.

I spent a total of eleven hours in the emergency room. During the blood transfusion, and after seeking permission from my nurse, I went for a stroll with my IV pole up to the third floor to visit my 3 East co-workers. It was around 11 p.m. and I knew they would be at the nurses' station checking their patients' medication administration records and chit-chatting. I sat at the nurses' station and visited for almost an hour. I looked dishevelled and grotesque in my stylish blue hospital gown, pink polka-dot pajama bottoms, and sky blue crocs; blood hanging from my IV pole and infusing down the long plastic tubing into my right arm; my abdomen extremely swollen; my legs resembling Polish sausages; my complexion still a little jaundiced, since I was only three weeks post-transplant. Not a picture of good health, but I knew my co-workers were used to seeing sick people. Nothing disgusting seems to bother us nurses. We can talking about nose mucous, vomit, and bloody stool over lunch and think nothing of it; it's like talking about the weather and politics. Out of curiosity, a few of my co-workers requested to see my stapled incision. I was bashful and a little reluctant to show off my forty-seven staples, but I pulled up my hospital gown—to my co-worker friends, it was fascinating to see what a liver transplant scar looks like.

On Monday morning, my parents brought the kids home. It was nice having them back; their constant energy and chaos brought some life back into the house. It was too quiet, and the house was unusually clean—I was used to stepping over toys and removing craft projects from the dining room table. The kids were overly excited to see me, but a little hesitant to give me a hug and kiss. They were afraid if they hugged me, they would break me. I initiated the hugs and hugged them tight with a side hug against my hip. Their little heads came up to the level of my incision, so I had to be careful. I let the kids kiss me on my cheek, and I cheek-kissed them back. Lip kisses were off limits, since kids carry germs. Watching Kyle and Sarah interact with me (snuggling next to me and touching my arms) and listening to them say, "I love you, Mommy," reinforced the fact that having the liver transplant was worth it—was worth the blood, pain, and disfigured abdomen. The kids will grow up with their mother, and I will be able to watch them grow up and raise families of their own.

I loved having the kids home, but I couldn't physically care for them. As a matter of fact, I couldn't even care for myself. Getting dressed and feeding myself was difficult - everything hurt. Sure, the kids were six and eight that summer and could dress and feed themselves, but they had more energy than I could handle. For the first week they were home, we sent them to day camps. Kevin was always home from work in time to help care for them in the evenings, and I was able to read stories and have movie nights with them. Then we enlisted the help of our thirteen-year-old neighbour as a babysitter for the next couple of weeks until they went back to school.

I was crossing my fingers that my hemoglobin would improve after my blood transfusion. During Tuesday's clinic appointment, Jill and Dr. Renner informed me that the transfusion did what it was supposed to do and had brought my hemoglobin up from sixty-two to ninety-six. *Thanks, blood donors, for saving my life.* This was the good news. The not-so-good news was that my creatinine hadn't gotten closer to being under ninety-seven and normal—it was up to 173. I guess my kidneys weren't too happy with the IV Lasix I was given. I was afraid I would require dialysis. Because of kidney failure, I was having trouble getting rid of the ascites. I left the hospital weighing 65.6 kilograms (144.3 pounds) and I still weighed the same two weeks later. I pleaded with Dr. Renner and Jill to tap me to quickly get rid of the excess fluid inside my abdomen. All this excess fluid was killing my back, abdomen, and legs, and making my life miserable. Dr. Renner agreed to a paracentesis to remove between four and seven litres of fluid from my abdomen. He recommended I find a local gastroenterologist to do the tap.

Kevin and I left the clinic appointment glad I was going to get some relief from my ascites. There is a long list of potential complications in the early post-transplant period: diabetes, wound infection, rejection episodes, and leg and abdominal swelling, to name a few. Ascites was by far the worst early post-transplant complication I experienced. If you have never experienced ascites, it is likely hard for you to understand how difficult it is to deal with. Imagine tying a sixteen kilograms (thirty-five pounds) bag of water around your abdomen and legs. Now try to do everyday activities. Try to bend forward and pick something up off the floor with water sloshing around inside your belly. Try walking on fat Flintstone feet that squish with each step and cramp. Try squeezing yourself into clothes that are so tight they leave seam indentations in your swollen flesh, if they fit at all. If you are a woman and have been pregnant, imagine going from your usual body weight to your pregnant self at nine months practically overnight. It is a shock to the body.

In my journal of my post-transplant days, I mention ascites often—how much it made life tough, and how it made me feel fat and hopeless. I had to go to Value Village and purchase a few pairs of maternity pants and shirts to bridge my wardrobe until I fit into my clothes again. I was kicking myself for donating my maternity clothes, although I never would have guessed I would need them again. But what gave me a sort-of odd appearance was the fact I had swollen legs and a belly that looked nine months pregnant, with bone-skinny arms, a flat chest, and a thin, sunken face. My unsightly appearance, coupled with my slow walking pace, unsteady gait, and use of a walker, drew public attention—and not the kind of attention I wanted. It hurt inside; it made me feel disgusting and self-conscious when people would point at me and snicker as they "quietly" commented about "the fat woman," or "the woman with something wrong." Little kids would point at me when we were at the park or in a store lineup, and would directly say to me, "You are fat," or whisper to their mothers, "That lady is fat." I hated the whispers, the comments, and the stares. It was all I could do to hold back tears or not yell at people, "I had a liver transplant! I'm not fat." I just tried to ignore *everything* negative. Deep down inside I was happy to be alive, and I didn't want my upbeat and positive bubble to burst. I tried to avoid the public most of the time—it was easier to just avoid the comments and stares.

The swelling also made it difficult to walk. Kevin liked to say, "Hurry up, Grandma." Walking from our house to our friends Andrea and Phil's house, only about one hundred meters down the street, was like walking a marathon in those early post-op days. My swollen thighs rubbed together and chafed. The swelling in my feet worsened when I stood up. My huge abdomen pulled on my back and caused back pain. I had to rent a four-wheel walker with a basket and seat; when it hurt too much to walk, I would sit for a break. I also needed the walker for balance. I was a little tippy because of muscle wasting. I felt like a newborn colt.

I wore compression stockings to help with circulation, keep fluid out of my feet and lower legs, and reduce the pain when I walked. I was used to wearing compression stockings because I wore them at work to help control the lower-leg swelling that commonly occurred while I was working a twelve-hour shift. Compression stockings kept my feet skinny enough to fit into my shoes. It was summer, and that meant it was hot and my legs were sweaty under those heavy nude-coloured stockings. I removed the knee-high stockings at night to wash them and wash my legs. I could take them off myself, but putting the stockings on each morning was a demanding task that required my husband's help. Applying the stockings made Kevin break out in a sweat. He had to squish my giant sausage legs into tight nylons—it was painful at times. Once the stockings were on, they didn't come off all day.

When my stockings were off, I took the opportunity to shower. Kevin had to assist me with the shower. Couples may shower together as a romantic affair, but having Kevin shower me was embarrassing. I did not want him to look at my bruised, swollen body held together with staples. I had trouble getting in and out of the tub and washing my feet, so Kevin reluctantly helped. I missed having a shower chair like in the hospital. I had to lean against the shower walls to avoid tipping over and slipping in the tub. When my legs were washed, long flakes of skin would slough off. My legs looked patchy with new skin and old skin, and the areas of new skin were so sensitive it felt like they had rug burn. Kevin once commented, "I didn't sign up to do this when I said 'I do.'" I replied, "We married in sickness and in health, so suck it up."

I had to keep my incision clean to help prevent infection. This meant I had to look at my staples as I cleansed them. There were several dime-sized scabs around the incision and a larger open area along my sternum, so I had to meticulously wash. No matter how often I looked at my incision, I always got that queasy, warm sensation inside. In my mind, I was always afraid I was going to burst open at the seams and my blood and guts would pour out. I blame my horrific thoughts on watching too many horror shows as a teen.

Every Tuesday I had my post-transplant clinic appointment at TGH with Dr. Renner. Because I wasn't allowed to drive for eight weeks after surgery, Kevin or my mom had to chauffeur me to my appointments. I booked my appointments first thing in the morning; being first usually meant less waiting because Dr. Renner was not behind in his schedule yet. However, it also meant fighting the morning rush-hour traffic on Highway 401 and that we had to leave Kitchener by 5:30 a.m. to make an 8 a.m. appointment.

I had the staples removed at my week-three and week-four clinic appointments. Half the staples were removed during the former, the other half during the latter. If all the staples had been removed at once, I might have fallen apart at the seams. I've removed staples from patients and they have never complain of it hurting, so I had the advantage of knowing what to expect and wasn't anxious or afraid. There is a nifty little tool that allows the nurse to bend the staples so they can be easily removed from the skin. The staples were left in for an extra week in one small section along my sternum that was stubborn to heal. When the nurse pulled out each staple, I could feel my skin pull—like the feeling of pulling out a sliver. I was still numb around my incision, so it didn't hurt, just a bit of a tug and a pinch.

The creepy thing wasn't the actual staple removal, but looking at the bloody dots on both sides of my incision afterwards. It looked like a sewing machine needle ran across my skin without being threaded. I had a row of little blood dots on each side of the incision—"railroad tracks" we sometimes call them. The nurse cleansed off the blood with white sterile gauze squares, and then placed a few clear plastic Steri-Strips over areas of my incision that were still slightly open. It felt good to have all forty-seven staples removed. I no longer had the pulling and pinching sensations along my incision, and I could wear clothes without having staples catch the fabric. I was far from being bikini ready, but at least I no longer looked like Frankenstein's monster.

Not too many people have seen my scar. Some of my co-workers have seen it, but that is because they are immune to all things medically disturbing and were intrigued to see what a liver transplant scar looks like. Of course, the transplant team has seen my scar. I even showed Dr. Winter because it isn't every day a patient walks into your family clinic and has a transplant scar to show. It was a teaching moment for Dr. Winter as far as I was concerned. When my son Kyle saw it, he commented, "It looks weird, Mommy, there are a whole bunch of lines. Sarah "accidentally" saw it when she was in my room one morning while I was dressing. Intrigued, she asked, "Mommy, is that where the doctors gave you your new liver?" I explained, "Yes, my new liver is inside me, and this is how the doctors put me back together."

My younger brother Bill saw it three months post-op. He later told me, "When I saw your scar, everything became too real. It was a glimpse of all of your pain and all of the people who invaded your person. That scar was hard to look at, Christine, it really was. You were like Humpty Dumpty . . . All of the men and all of the women helped to put Christine back together again." What really made me see my scar in a different light was when Bill told me, "That scar made me happy. You got into a fight and won! It's a battle wound." I guess I did win a battle. I won my battle over liver disease, and my scar is proof I survived. Maybe I should wear it proudly like a badge of honour, since it is a mark of strength and perseverance. I highly doubt I will go so far as to describe my scar as *beautiful* or *sexy*. But I will say, I have become "used to" seeing it after living with it for one year now. It has become part of who I am and will be my permanent, unique branding to show I am a liver transplant survivor.

My husband hasn't seen it. Why? He says he doesn't want that image in his head. Some people aren't comfortable looking at scars. He doesn't like anything medical. Plus, I'm not one to just flip up my shirt and say, "Hey, do you want to see my scar?" It was a necessity to keep me alive, not something I feel I need to go around flaunting. I have even gone so far as to keep the lights off or to wear lingerie to cover the scar during intimate moments. I'm sure Kevin will come across my scar someday, when he is ready to see it and I feel comfortable enough to do the big reveal. *Maybe by then, my scar will be a little sexy.* I was thinking of blending the scar into a peace-sign tattoo. But come to think of it, tattoos involve needles, so that isn't really a good idea.

I had some pretty high expectations post-transplant. I expected my life to return to "normal" quite quickly after returning home. It made me feel angry and let down when Dr. Renner and Jill informed me, during one of my clinic appointments, that my ALP liver enzyme was significantly elevated—another of the post-transplant complications. Normal ALP is 44 to 147 IU/L, and my lab value was 458. I knew I was faced with the now very real, and ever–present, threat that my own body will endure complications or reject the grafted liver. A high ALP was by no means a rejection or return of my disease, but it did suggest that there was a problem with my bile ducts. It is possible post-transplant to develop narrowing in the bile ducts, especially where the ducts are connected to the bile ducts of the new liver. This narrowing can cause a reduced flow of bile from the liver into the small bowel and may lead to liver inflammation. To treat this problem, either the medication ursodiol is given to dissolve cholesterol and thin the bile, or a stent is placed into the bile duct to try to widen the duct opening.

Before doing any invasive procedures, Dr. Renner decided to just "watch and wait" my high ALP and see if it would trend down on its own. When it remained elevated for a month, Dr. Renner said we needed to find the cause and perhaps correct the issue. But an ultrasound at TGH revealed nothing significant, and my bile ducts appeared unobstructed. *Phew . . . nothing to warrant cutting open my body again.*

It is important to keep all the liver enzymes within normal limits to prevent the new liver from becoming inflamed or damaged. My ALP continued to be abnormal, but why? Dr. Renner ordered a specialized MRI called a magnetic resonance cholangiopancreatography (MRCP) to image my biliary tree. I had two MRCP tests, one at Grand River Hospital in Kitchener and one at Toronto Western Hospital. The gastroenterologist who reviewed my MRCPs said that "there might possibly be a stricture or narrowing in the right hepatic duct" but didn't feel this possible narrowing warranted an ERCP (a type of endoscopy to help diagnose and treat problems associated with the bile ducts and pancreatic ducts). Thank goodness, because that procedure involved yet another needle, and frankly, I was tired of needles and hospitals.

A liver biopsy can also be used to help determine the cause of an elevated ALP. When Dr. Renner and Jill first mentioned a liver biopsy, it sent chills through my body and made me panic. The thought of that ginormous needle penetrating my scarred abdomen and new liver was terrifying. Besides, I had so much fluid in my abdomen, how was the radiologist going to penetrate my skin without me springing a leak? Dr. Renner answered that very question with, "We will have to do a transvenous liver biopsy." Now I was really upset and scared. A biopsy through my abdomen was something I didn't like; a transvenous biopsy was something I dreaded. It involves inserting a long catheter through a vein in the neck into the hepatic vein and directly into the liver to obtain a tissue sample. *Just writing about this procedure is giving me the creeps.* Dr. Renner insisted on a liver biopsy because he wanted to gather information regarding the cause of my elevated ALP as well as gain insight about why I was having difficulty with ascites.

If you have ever been booked for a medical test such as an MRI, CT scan, or biopsy, you know appointments are booked a few months out. Luckily, this delay gave me some time to have two abdominal taps prior to the biopsy—meaning, to my great relief, that I lost enough abdominal fluid to have a percutaneous liver biopsy through my abdomen and didn't have to have a catheter inserted into my neck after all.

My first tap was on Wednesday, August 14, with Dr. Golubov. He was the same gastroenterologist assigned to me at St. Mary's Hospital before the transplant. Running into Dr. Golubov again allowed me to properly thank him for such great care. When Dr. Golubov inserted the plastic catheter into my abdomen, blood-tinged fluid immediately began draining into the urinary bag hanging on the side of the gurney. The fluid should have been a whitish-yellow colour, but it was blood-tinged from the trauma I endured during surgery. The catheter was removed after seven litres of fluid was drained. Litre by litre, I could practically see my abdomen shrinking like a balloon deflating. I had some abdominal cramping, but no pain (I took Percocet beforehand). I was given IV albumin after the tap to reduce the incidence of circulatory dysfunction such as a low blood volume and low blood pressure. Albumin consists of proteins found in human blood—a kind stranger donated the albumin when he or she donated blood.

In a matter of four hours, I lost almost fourteen pounds. *I think I've found the secret to weight loss—screw those diet pills!* Even my mood was instantly lighter after losing the fluid. It was like I was at happy hour at a bar, ironically. But there was one problem (there always seems to be a problem): my back went into some horrible spasms. All the ascites had kept a constant pressure on my back muscles, and they had become accustomed to being strained and pulled on. Without the added weight pulling on my back, I experienced intermittent sharp, quivering spasms through my spine, from my tailbone to my neck. The only way to lessen the pain was to hold still and let the spasms subside while panting like a dog—it worked!

Dr. Renner was hoping my kidney function would improve and help eliminate more fluid. Unfortunately, those darn old kidneys refused to help me out. I couldn't take Lasix because my creatinine was in the 160 range. Despite the tap, I continued to have complications from the ascites. My lady parts were so swollen that it hurt to walk or stand for long periods of time. My legs were still Polish sausages, and my thighs rubbed together and chafed. My belly (and hernia) protruded outward, and fluid sloshed around inside me like the ocean during a storm. My children were embarrassed to have me pick them up from school because their friends would ask them what was wrong with their mom. I couldn't even get down to the floor to play with the kids. Everything hurt, nothing was easy, and I wasn't living the "normal life" I had envisioned. I was losing patience, and finally, I broke down. I cried like I hadn't cried in a long time. I wanted to shut myself in my bedroom and never face the world again. I'd tried to stay positive after my transplant. I was so happy to be alive. But why did receiving a life-saving transplant have to mean living like this?

I knew if I lost the remainder of the fluid, I could combat the depression that was beginning to take hold. I knew wholeheartedly that losing the fluid meant I could live a "normal life" again. Jill informed me that Dr. Renner was willing to try twenty milligrams of Lasix for three days—a small dose, but at least it was something. Jill advised me to have my kidney function checked in three days. I did what I was told, and wouldn't you know it, my kidneys weren't happy with the Lasix and my creatinine increased. But I did lose 5.8 pounds in those three days and felt better about myself.

On Monday, September 16, Dr. Renner agreed to another paracentesis, likely because I bugged him enough to let me be tapped again. Actually, he agreed because I had kept off the fluid from the first tap and didn't develop an infection. This time, I didn't take a Percocet because I was trying to wean myself off it—the opiates were making me live in a haze and causing some bizarre and scary dreams—so during the tap, the abdominal cramps were uncomfortable.

After the four-hour tap, I had lost another 7.8 litres of fluid, which equates to 17.2 pounds. As my nurse struggled to carry the two urinary bags of fluid to the dirty utility closet, she yelled back at me, "I'm carrying your water-baby twins." I now weighed 50.2

kilograms (110.4 pounds), less than I did when I rowed flyweight in high school. Underneath all that weight was truly my slim self. What made me smile and giggle was when Kevin assisted me into the passenger seat of our Pontiac Vibe and I could comfortably put on the seat belt without adjusting it under my protruding abdomen.

When I arrived home, I examined my new body in the bedroom mirror. I didn't recognize myself: a stick figure with a peace-sign scar. Attractive I was not! I really noticed my umbilical hernia now, and it was even more painful. I purchased a few pairs of high-waisted Spanx underwear to help push in my hernia and provide support to my weak abdominal muscles. I also purchased soft Lycra sports bras with padding to give my flat chest some breasts. My bras dug into my incision, so I had to find ones that were a tube style. My incision runs along my sternum and begins between my breasts—the surgeons were male and likely thought nothing of placing the incision at the bust line.

The night after my second tap, I had the soundest sleep. I didn't have to sleep in a pillow tower. I could sleep on my side or back without any discomfort. This meant Kevin could sleep next to me again. Having Kevin back in bed meant I could snuggle up next to him and keep warm.

The umbilical hernia continued to protrude outward and reminded me of my belly button when I was pregnant. It caused sharp pains if I bent sideways the wrong way or sat up quickly. I constantly pushed it in with my index finger when it stuck out. I was concerned and wanted to get a surgeon's opinion regarding whether I should have umbilical hernia repair. Dr. Renner referred me to Dr. Markus Selzner, an abdominal transplant surgeon at TGH, who said my hernia was small and therefore he wouldn't recommend surgery. Surgery would require him to make a long incision down my abdomen, and post-op recovery is upwards of three months. I couldn't put my life on hold for another three months. I wanted to bike again and return to work. Dr. Selzner recommended I keep my weight under control. If I keep a flat abdomen, the hernia is less likely to protrude outward. He also suggested that I keep my abdominal muscles strong by doing isometric abdominal exercises such as planks. I find wearing Spanx underwear or my pregnancy belt also helps—anything to avoid being butchered again.

From September 16 onward, I felt I could eat whatever I wanted. I needed to gain weight. At 110.4 pounds, I had twenty-two pounds to go before returning to my "normal" weight. I don't like being really skinny because it makes me look unhealthy—my bones show, my face is sunken, and I am physically weak. I like a little meat on my bones. I still had to follow a low-sodium diet so I wouldn't gain the fluid back, but I was able to put away the blood glucose supplies because my sugars were well controlled—no more finger sticks. That meant I could increase the amount of carbohydrates I consumed. Instead of half a banana, I could scarf down a whole banana. For the first time in my life, I didn't have to watch my figure. Food was a free-for-all. It was like being at an all-you-can-eat buffet every day. When I baked chocolate chip cookies, I didn't just stop at one, I ate at least a dozen without feeling guilty.

To prevent myself from gaining too much weight too quickly, I exercised. I walked a lot, initially with my walker and then on my own. Thankfully, I had my transplant in the summer, so I didn't have to dodge snowbanks and watch out for ice patches. I also enrolled in a total-body workout class that promised to be a combination of cardio, strength, and flexibility training to improve strength and stamina. I figured the class was a good fit because I had *no* strength or stamina at this point. Those first few classes kicked my butt. I wasn't able to keep up, so I worked at my own pace and the instructor provided alternative exercises. I was slower than most of the seniors in the class, and I had to accept that. After stretching and relaxation exercises at the end of class, I found it tricky to get off the mat. In fact, during the first class I actually couldn't roll up on my own, and one of the participants had to assist me. Some participants asked if I was ill or recovering from surgery. I certainly didn't jump around and move like Mick Jagger.

The seniors were more agile than I was until halfway through the fall semester, when my muscles built themselves back up. It felt good when I could do jumping jacks again and not get stuck down on the mat. The instructor told me she was proud to see such an improvement in my fitness.

I also took up swimming laps once my incision healed. Before I could go swimming, though, I had to purchase a one-piece bathing suit. Up until now, I had worn only bikinis, but I wasn't quite ready to show off my peace-sign scar to the public. I found a one-piece with bright tropical flowers splattered across it. It was definitely not my style and I felt like I was wearing a body glove. The swimsuit also had a built-in bra with cups that gave me fake boobs. That part was much appreciated.

Rockin' my new swimsuit, I took it easy and used a flutter board to swim fifty meters. I was used to swimming over thirty laps at a time, but now even a couple laps was a workout. *Geez, what happened to my strength?* Having "warmed up," I donned my Speedo goggles and attempted to swim a breaststroke. I say *attempted*, but what I mean is, I nearly drowned. My legs and arms didn't have the strength I expected of them. I made it from the shallow end to about halfway across the deep end, and then had to frantically tread water and doggy-paddle in an effort to make it to the poolside. I went under the water a few times as I struggled to keep my head up. *Are the lifeguards going to come rescue me? Can't they see I'm drowning?* An elderly lady gabbing with her friend in the deep end was sitting on a pool noodle, leisurely paddling. She saw me struggling and whipped her pool noodle toward my arms. I grabbed hold and slowly kicked my way over to the side. I thanked her for saving my life. She didn't speak English, but smiled as if to say, "You're welcome." I survived a liver transplant but nearly drowned in my local public pool. I stuck to the shallow end after that and found some dumbbell water weights to play with.

With the kids back at school, they brought home germs—creepy, crawly, microscopic germs that made someone who is immunocompromised, like myself, sick all the time. Knowing that little kids are germ carriers, I made my kids, and their friends, wash their hands as soon as they came home from school—a squirt or two of antibacterial hand sanitizer, then they could play. I was paranoid that they were going to bring home a disease that would send me packing my bags for another hospitalization. Late in September, one of my little germ carriers got me sick with a cold. The cold spread throughout our house, so there was no way I could avoid it—gloves, mask, extra hand-sanitizer wouldn't have helped. Kevin, Kyle, and Sarah had the sniffles for a few days. But not me. I was sick for three weeks and developed a nasty congested cough along with a runny nose. I left a message for Jill asking if there was anything I could take. I had been advised not to take decongestants post-transplant because they can increase blood pressure and harm the liver. Jill called me back and advised me to take a saline mist nasal spray for my blocked nose. She did give me permission to take the narcotic Hycodan as needed, to help control my cough—which I did, along with other cold-treatment strategies like VapoRub and a vaporizer. Just when I got better, another germ-carrying child of mine got me sick again with another cold. This time the dang cold lasted for one month. I had three severe colds between the beginning of the school year and Christmas. The joys of being immunocompromised!

On December 23, I received some wonderful news: *all* of my liver enzymes were normal. *Normal*, what's that? I hadn't had normal enzymes since I don't know when. Even the ALP was normal. "Watch and wait" had worked, and I avoided an ERCP or taking additional meds. My body smartened itself up like I had kept telling it to. With all my liver enzymes normalized, Dr. Renner stopped my prednisone. I had been on prednisone since 1987, when I was thirteen-years-old. I was a little skeptical that this medication would be stopped for good. My body likes prednisone. Every time a doctor tries to discontinue prednisone, my liver enzymes rise. I suspected this would be a temporary medication change, and I was right. In February 2014, I was put back on twenty milligrams of prednisone for a small rejection or possible return of my disease.

Transplants change people, not only physically but psychologically. I've heard recipients call the psychological effects "transplant remorse." I know I experienced transplant remorse, and still do. It is so heartbreaking to know that someone died, and that their family and friends are out there grieving the loss of their loved one, while I get to continue living life. I get to live the happy side of the organ transplant story, while the donor family lives the sad side. I wake up every day and thank God I am alive and get to spend another day with my family and friends. The donor's family wakes up every day and misses and thinks of their loved one. They only have memories left. It isn't fair that they have to suffer. It just isn't fair. And that's what bothers me and brings so much heartache—knowing the donor family is out there suffering as they mourn the loss of their son or daughter, sister or brother. Why does it have to be this way?

I know I didn't cause this stranger's death by needing a new liver. But knowing I have a dead stranger's liver inside me is eerie. *Does this person watch me from heaven to see if I am taking good care of his or her liver?* I think of the donor every day. I wonder if he or she knew, when registering to become an organ donor, that he or she would actually become a donor—likely not. I wish I knew who my donor was because I share a special bond with him or her. My donor's liver is keeping me alive. I wish I could associate a real person with my donor liver, for peace of mind. Was my donor young and male? I'm pretty sure yes. I tried to listen to subtle things the transplant team said in the operating room before I was put under. The liver was "biggish," and the resident said, "The liver is young and healthy." But one of the questions I would like answered more than anything is, *How did he die? Was his death from a disease? Was he involved in a fatal car accident* (which is my inkling)? *Did he die in a drowning or natural disaster?* Anything is possible. But knowing that he was young, he was likely involved in a car accident. I could be way off. I am not sure I'll ever find out the true identity of my donor and how he died. And if I don't find out the answers to my questions, I will just have to accept this as one of life's unknowns.

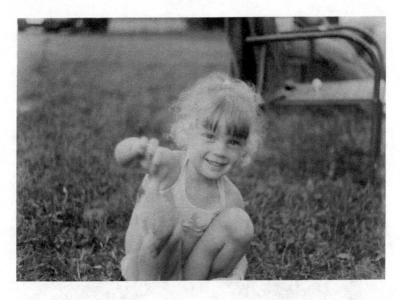

3 years old – caught my first fish

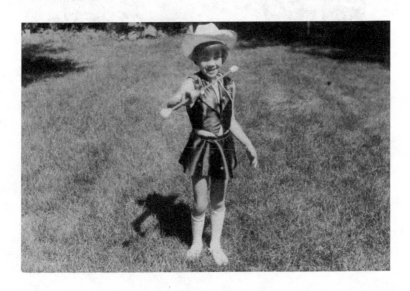

7 years old – I was a majorette

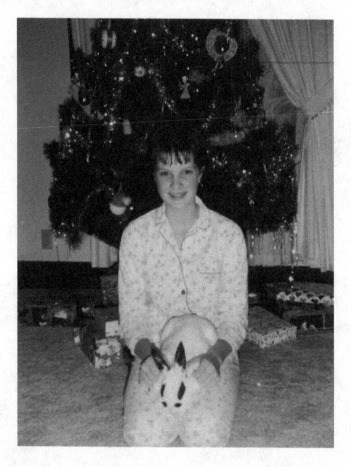

With my pet rabbit Bandit

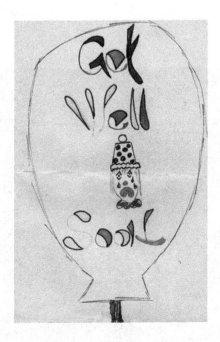

The card my grade 8 class made. My classmates signed the inside

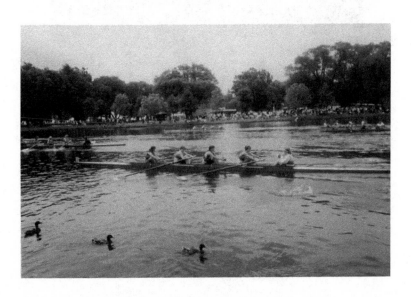

Lightweight 4 – Centre Island Rowing Regatta

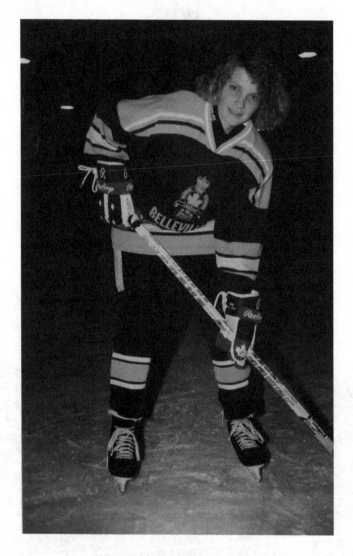

16 years old – Belleville girls hockey

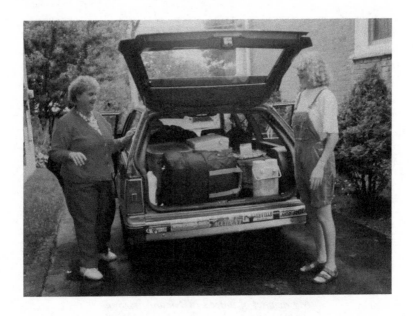

Moving to Vancouver Island with Grandma

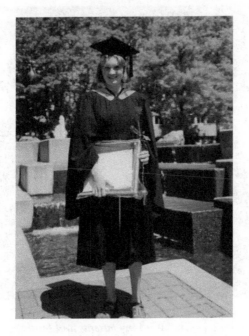

Graduation from the University of Victoria

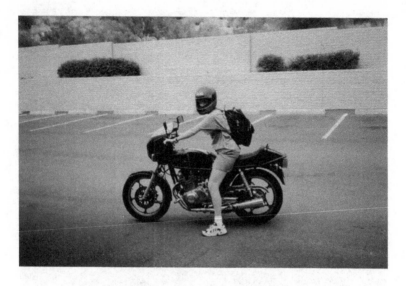

My new set of wheels in Tucson Arizona

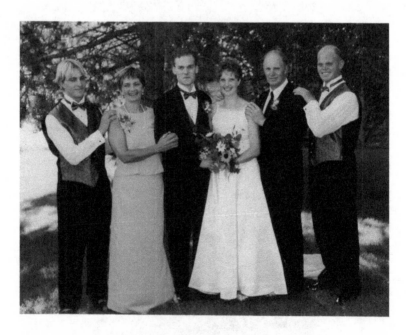

Our wedding. With my parents and brothers.
Bill on the left & Andy on the right

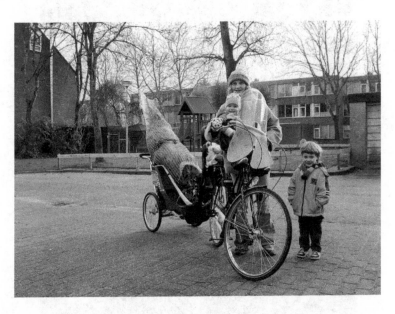

I biked everywhere and could carry just about anything on my bike

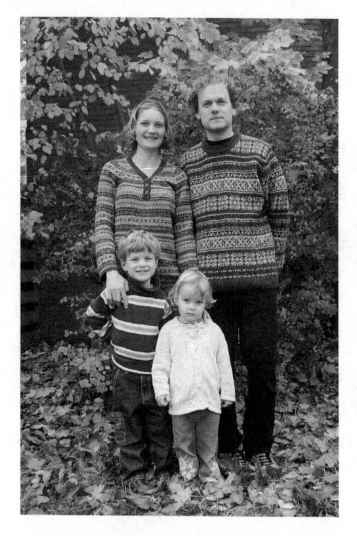

Family photograph in Groningen

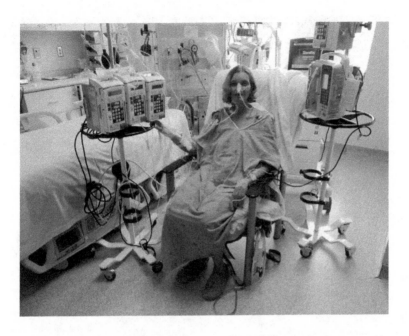

Post op day 1 in the ICU

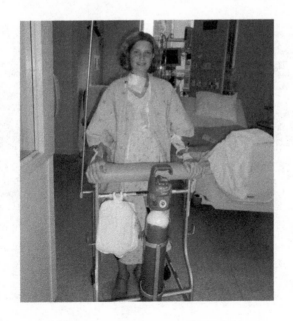

Post op day 3 in Step Down

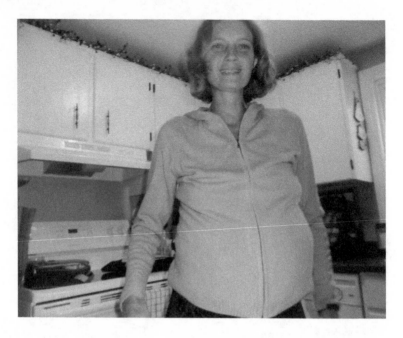

7 weeks post op – me with my fluid-filled abdomen

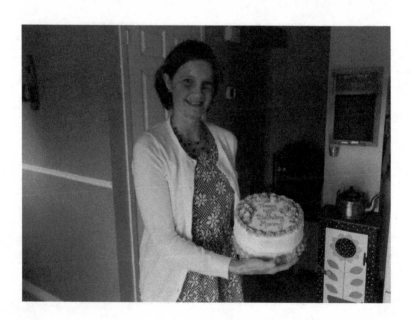

March 24, 2013 – Made it to my 40ᵗʰ birthday

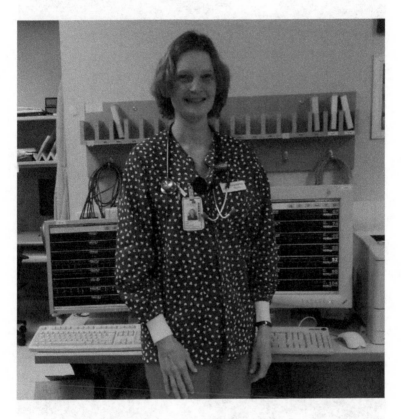

Return to work on 3 East Cardiology

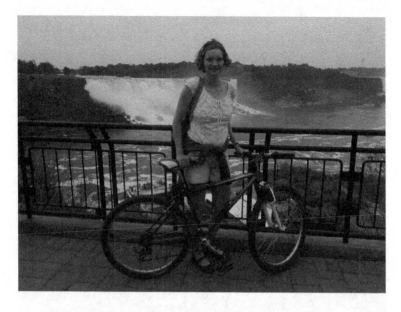

*10 months post op – Biked 44 km from Niagara-
on-the-Lake to Niagara Falls and back*

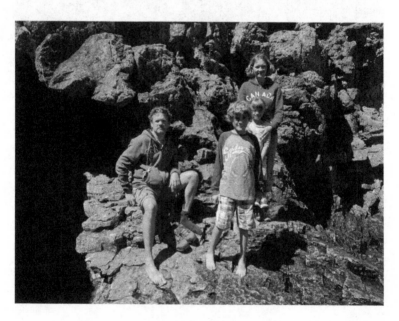

Family photograph August 2014

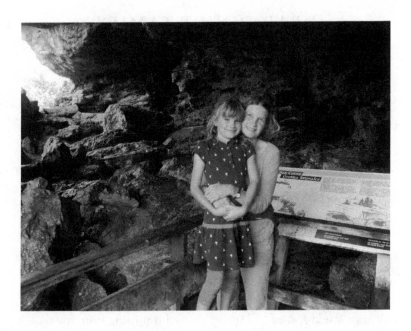

With 7 year old Sarah

Chapter 20

DEAR DONOR FAMILY

My life goes on because of my donor and his or her family. And the donor's "life" goes on inside me, and inside other recipients who received his or her organs. The donor's life is not the same, though. The donor is not the same bubbly, artistic preteen, or the same respected and well-loved father; sadly, he or she is no longer with us in that capacity. I feel I share a special bond with my donor. My donor's liver is able to live inside me and continues giving me life. I am not sure how other recipients feel, but personally, I wish I knew for sure who my donor was. Knowing my donor's identity would sort of "fill in" what I feel is missing from my transplant story. I want to carry an image of my donor in my mind, along with the already precious gift inside my abdomen.

The Trillium Gift of Life Network sends a letter to the families of donors, thanking them for their donation and informing them of the outcome. Letters from recipients are also forwarded to donor families through TGLN. All recipients are encouraged to write a thank-you letter to their donor family. Some recipients write more than once, and some do not write at all. The letter is a sincere way to thank the anonymous donor family for their choice and generosity, and it is often helpful in the psychological healing process—at least it was for me. For most recipients, the problem with writing the letter is not with *wanting* to write the letter, but with knowing just what to say. Recipients often feel *thank you* is not enough and struggle over the right words to express their heartfelt gratitude.

Janine is the daughter of a donor. Her father's organs were donated. I met her through the Life Donation Awareness Association (LDAA—you can read more about the association and Janine's story in the final part of this book). I asked Janine if her family received any correspondence from her dad's recipients. She shared with me, "We know what TGLN told us at the time, which was that three middle-aged males received my dad's organs. One man received my dad's liver, and two other men received a kidney each. I'm not sure why we never received any letters—it's not something I dwell on really. We didn't donate (on behalf of my dad) with expectations. We donated because it felt like the right thing to do."

After joining the LDAA group a year after her dad passed away, Janine volunteered at a BeADonor booth at St. Mary's Hospital along with liver recipient Bob. Bob reminded Janine of everything she'd thought her dad's recipients might be like in age, appearance, and maybe even personality. Janine told me, "As Bob and I talked about our stories, he explained that it was hard for him to begin to write a letter to his donor family. It was particularly difficult because nothing seemed 'good enough' or 'right' when he wrote it down, so he had never actually completed the process. Bob told me how he'd struggled with the guilt of knowing someone died so he could live, and he expressed concern that if or when he reached out to his donor family, he may be opening up raw wounds for them. That conversation shed a lot of light on how 'the other side' feels post-transplant. I could see the sadness in Bob's eyes; we really connected that evening.

"Bob asked me what I would like to hear about if my dad's recipient(s) ever wrote to us. My answer was simple. 'Just that they are okay and that they are living life to the fullest. Just the simple stuff really.' I explained to Bob that for me, the donation was a part of, but not definitive of, my dad's death. Losing him was the hardest part, and everything else that happened after allowed us to make the proverbial lemonade from lemons.

"I never expected anything from our recipient(s) or their families then, nor do I now. I guess it's because I had sort of figured that perhaps those men might be a bit like my dad, meaning they were middle-aged men who may find being "sappy," sharing feelings and being emotional, a bit difficult at the best of times, let alone post-transplant. My conversation with Bob sort of confirmed my headspace. Everything Bob said to me was exactly what I felt my dad's recipients might have felt."[2]

For me, writing to the donor family was both challenging and therapeutic. Like many transplant recipients, I battled with guilt surrounding my transplant. When I prayed for a liver to become available in time to save my life, I felt like I was praying for God to allow someone to die so I could live. I felt guilty knowing that someone accidentally died July 20 (or around that date), and if it weren't for his or her unfortunate death, I would not have received a new liver. Nurse friends have told me that the donor would have died regardless of my need for a liver, and it is by chance that the donor's liver was a match and able to save my life.

I felt compelled to thank the family for their decision to donate, and for honouring their loved one's wish to be a donor. I wanted the letter to be heartfelt and sincere. I had been thinking in my early weeks of recovery about what I was going to say to my donor family, and I had gone through many scenarios in my head. What if they did not want to hear from me? How do I say I am happy I got this liver without making it sound like I am happy their loved one passed away? What if I did not get a response from them? How would I feel then?

---

2   Since the time of writing, Bob has written to his donor family.

It took me weeks to complete the letter because I would write a sentence and start crying. Most of the letter was written while my eyes were blurry from tears. How could I possibly thank someone for giving me the gift of life? Allowing my children to grow up with a mother . . . my husband with a wife . . . my parents with a daughter.

I would like to share my letter, as I truly appreciate the courage and strength it took for the donor family to make their life-saving decision to donate.

September 10, 2013

Dear Donor Family,

It is nearly seven weeks since I received your family's gift of life. I am so sorry for the loss of your loved one. I know it must be difficult to live without him/her. I hope you can find comfort knowing that your loved one was able to donate their liver, giving me a second chance at life.

I am thirty-nine-years-old, a mother and a wife. I have two children; my son is eight and my daughter is six. When I was thirteen-years-old, I developed chronic autoimmune hepatitis. It remains unknown as to why I developed this particular disease. Up until the July long weekend, I was able to manage the disease with medications and lived a fairly normal life. I was cycling, playing with my kids, working nearly full time, and doing home renovations. I suddenly became very sick and was hospitalized. My liver and kidneys quickly began to fail and I needed a liver transplant to live. I was put on the transplant list and received a liver transplant from your loved one, two days later, on July 21st. The ironic thing is July 21st is also my daughter's birthday. Now every year we can celebrate her birthday and my new life.

I am a registered nurse and work in the cardiac unit at an Ontario hospital. I really enjoy being a nurse and helping patients with heart disease. I plan on using my nursing background and my experience as a transplant recipient to educate others on the importance of the gift of life.

Recovery has not been easy, but I keep reminding myself that I am still alive and will do everything possible to live a normal and healthy life thanks to your donation. Since receiving my new liver, I have been able to take my children to their first day of school this year. I was able to celebrate my thirteenth anniversary with my husband.

I often wonder whom it is that I share a special bond with; who is the person whose liver is inside me? If you feel comfortable contacting me, please do. I would like to know more about your loved one. If you would like to remain anonymous, I truly understand.

Without your donation, I would not have been able to remain a part of such a wonderful family. It is nice to be able to watch my children grow up with a mother. And, it is nice to spend time with my parents, brothers, and the rest of my extended family.

I know that no words I would possibly say could heal you from the grief of your overwhelming loss, please accept my deepest heartfelt sympathy. I will cherish your family's gift for the rest of my life.

Thank you,

The Recipient

My letter was submitted in an unsealed envelope to my transplant coordinator, Jill Quance, on September 17. Jill forwarded the letter to TGLN. Letters are reviewed before being mailed to ensure they remain anonymous. Under the Human Tissue Gift Act, the Government of Ontario requires that both the recipient's and the donor's identities remain confidential. For this reason, the transplant team asks that the letter not contain personal information such as names, residence, workplace, or religious affiliation.

Despite the mandatory confidentiality, with the power of the Internet it's possible to search online for potential donors. How many of us recipients google accidents or obituaries that may fit with the timing of transplant? It is tempting to play detective and try and figure out who the donor may have been.

Just as recipients look for their donors, some donor families search for the recipients online and in newspapers, or sometimes, donor families and recipients happen to find each other at an organ donation event. Some donor families write back and even form a bond with recipients. These are the only ways the true identity of the donor and nature of the death are revealed—if the donor and recipient discover each other's identities and connect, or if the donor family sends correspondence to the recipient through TGLN.

TGLN staff have told me most transplant recipients do not hear from their donor families. "Many donor families are overwhelmed with emotion and may have difficulty expressing themselves. Some may respond to your letter, while others may make the choice not to write. Remember that the donor family may still be coping with the loss of their loved one, and people deal with grief in different ways. While you are celebrating your renewed health, your donor family is dealing with their loss." I was also told that, sadly, sometimes the donor letter is returned if the family moved and did not provide TGLN with their new address.

In addition to sending donor families a letter informing them of the outcome of their gift of donation (regardless of whether the family receives any letters from recipients), TGLN also offers a donor-family support program. The relationship between the TGLN Family Services advisor and the donor family begins when consent to donate is given. The Donor Family Support program continues over the twelve months following donation. This relationship with TGLN may continue beyond that time; for example, through volunteer work.

Every donor family is invited to the yearly Celebration of Life event hosted by TGLN, to acknowledge and celebrate the gift of donation. The event is held in cities across Ontario. Donor families are encouraged to attend within eighteen months of their donation, as a way to help them heal. A transplant recipient speaks at the event, on behalf of all recipients, to give thanks to donor families and show them that organ donation really does make a difference and allows a person to continue to live a normal, healthy life. The Trillium Gift of Life Network's Donor Memorial Quilt also travels across Ontario and is displayed at each Celebration of Life event. The quilt is one of the ways donor families can honour their loved ones: families and friends create a quilt patch with photos, symbols, special words, and information about their loved one.

I think of my donor family every day because I am reminded several times a day of my liver transplant: the scar I see when I dress, the continual tight feeling around my abdomen, the 9 a.m. and 9 p.m. medication schedule, the frequent doctor's appointments, and the fact that I am alive. I am thankful for all donor families—you are true heroes!

As an organ and tissue coordinator at TGLN posted, "I am in continual amazement at how people—even in their saddest moments—think of others. Whether it's honouring a loved one's choice to donate their organs, or thinking of the recipients themselves, I am always awed at how people move beyond their own devastation to care about others."

Chapter 21

MY OLD LIVER IN A PICKLE JAR

My inquisitive eight-year-old son asked what happened to my old liver. That was an excellent question. *Where was my old liver?* I hadn't wondered about it; it's funny what kids think of. In a pickle jar downstairs in a hospital lab, labelled *surgical waste*, according to the transplant team. They didn't quite say "pickle jar," but that's how I imagined it. The team told me that this was probably the first time they had been asked that question. *Inquisitive minds want to know.*

I really wanted to see my old cirrhotic liver, but that could not be arranged. I had an image in my head of what it looked like from googling pictures on the Internet. It was likely hard, lumpy and bumpy, small and stiff, and dark brownish-red.

During my first visit to the post-transplant clinic, I was given the surgical pathology report on my old liver. Being the curious nurse I am, I was excited to read about my old liver. I know, maybe I'm a little odd, but my old liver was part of me for thirty-nine years. It was a bittersweet farewell to an old friend. It kept me living for a long time before it retired.

Except the surgical pathology report revealed that my old liver hadn't retired—more like it had kicked the bucket. Reading the report was a little frightening. The transplant surgeon, Dr. David Grant, who spoke with my mom was right. I had likely had only a couple days left to live. Fibrosis (thickening and scarring of connective tissue) was at a stage four out of four. Early stages of liver fibrosis (stages one and two) are reversible. Stage four is indicative of severe liver cirrhosis, permanent scarring, and problematic and irreversible changes in the structure of the liver. The liver is a unique organ because it has the ability to regenerate, to replace damaged liver cells with healthy ones. But with liver cirrhosis, the liver can no longer replace those damaged cells, and they continue to build up over many years, making the liver hard and nodular (lumpy and bumpy). From ages thirteen to thirty-nine, my liver was chronically inflamed. Chronic inflammation continually caused liver cell damage, which increased the growth of fibrous tissue in my liver.

There were no gross abnormalities noted, meaning there were no tumours or strange growths found on my old liver. My history of autoimmune hepatitis was noted, not surprisingly. My whole liver was atrophic, decreased in size. Severe cholestasis was one of the main features found in my liver tissue. Cholestasis occurs when bile cannot flow properly from the gallbladder to the small intestine to help break down food for digestion. Cholestasis is what gave me a jaundiced appearance, as well as pale grey bowel movements, dark urine, and occasional bouts of abdominal pain.

My gallbladder joined my old liver as "surgical waste." It was also removed, as promised, during my liver transplant. My gallbladder was nothing but trouble; I didn't need it anyway. What I thought was interesting was there were no gallstones noted. My pre-transplant ultrasounds and medical imaging studies showed the presence of gallstones—not to mention the intense pain I'd suffered that had been attributed to them. *Where did the gallstones go?*

I have tucked away my surgical pathology report in a box among the pile of other medical reports I have accumulated over the years. If I miss my old liver, I can always go back and read about it. *Farwell old friend ... We knew each other our whole lives, but it was time for you to be replaced.*

Chapter 22

RESEARCH OPPORTUNITIES

Toronto General Hospital is well known for its groundbreaking research. Organ transplants are based on research in TGH's laboratories and clinics. Bulletin boards outside hospital elevators are cluttered with volunteer opportunities for research studies.

The first study I volunteered for was for the Liver Transplant Biobank Registry. Dr. Gary Yu approached me while I was still in the transplant unit, seven days post-op. I listened to what Dr. Yu had to say about the study. He explained that when a person receives an organ from a donor, the recipient's immune system may think the new organ is a foreign object because the recipient's immune system detects that the antigens on the cells of the new organ are different, or not "matched." Mismatched organs, or organs that are not matched closely enough, can trigger a transplant rejection. To help prevent a rejection, doctors try to closely match the donor organ to the recipient. The more similar the antigens are between the donor and recipient, the less likely that the organ will be rejected.

I consented to the study because I want to help researchers in organ transplantation and they need volunteers like me. Without volunteers there would be no study. My commitment was to donate a small amount of blood on days seven, fourteen, and thirty, and then six months and annually after transplant. (I like how the information sheet says "a small amount of blood." Six vials is not a small amount. Instead of an extra lab draw, I scheduled my blood samples at the same time as clinic lab draws. One needle stick is all I can handle!)

The Liver Transplant Biobank Registry is a research program to collect and store, for future research, human biological samples (blood and biopsy tissue) from individuals who have received or may receive an organ transplant. The collected biological specimens are intended to be used in future studies to help identify genes and/or molecules that play a key role in the regulation of immune rejection. Basically, the study's objective is to figure out why some people have a transplant rejection, while others do not. If the cause of rejection can be identified, new remedies and medications with higher efficiency and fewer side effects can be formulated.

During my first post-transplant appointment, I was approached to participate in another study, "Epidemiology and Economic Evaluation of Surgical Site Infections after Liver Transplant." This fancy title translates into a research study that is looking at how often, and why, surgical site infections occur in recipients following a liver transplant. The research information sheets handed to me stated: "Following surgery, some patients may develop infection at the site of incision in spite of preventative measures. Organisms (bacteria or fungi) usually identified at the infected site are commonly found on the skin and in the intestines. All transplant patients are given antibiotics, so initially experts did not believe that surgical site infections were an important problem. Recent research, however, has found that surgical site infections may harm the transplanted organ, and they can also affect patient survival."

My only commitment was to allow Dr. Renner to assess my incisional site at transplant clinic visits. No needle stick required—that's my kind of study. Fortunately, I did not experience an infection, so my participation in the study was minimal. The research team was interested in those patients with an incisional infection.

The third study was mailed to me by Dr. Angela Cheung at the Francis Family Liver Clinic at Toronto Western Hospital. This study is investigating "The Impact of Autoimmune Liver Disease on Fertility and Pregnancy." It is believed that in some women, autoimmune liver disease has an impact on pregnancy, and in others, pregnancy may have an impact on autoimmune liver disease. The study's goal is to determine what effects autoimmune liver disease has on fertility and during pregnancy, in both mother and baby. When I was contemplating becoming pregnant, ten years ago now, I wish I could have had access to the results of a study like this one. There were so many unknowns at the time, and Dr. Heathcote and Dr. Morrero reiterated what I already knew, that pregnancy was possible but risky. I had lived with autoimmune hepatitis for seventeen years at that point, but was otherwise healthy; my liver was not found to be cirrhotic yet, and I was taking prednisone and Imuran, which were not category X meds (meds with the highest potential to cause birth defects).

My commitment to this study was to complete an in-depth survey on my gynecological history as well as my pregnancy history. I shared many intimate details, such as how our children were conceived, my monthly cycles, complications during pregnancy, the health of our children, and information on my disease postnatal. I had to dig through archived medical notes from Michigan and the Netherlands to provide accurate details. With so many personal questions asked, I chuckled at the statement under risks: "There is a potential for the survey questions to cause emotional discomfort due to their personal nature. You may skip any questions should you feel uncomfortable answering."

Participating in these studies brought back memories of my student days in the biology labs at UVic. I hope to have access to the results of these studies someday, but like many studies, it takes years to gather the data before the article can be written.

Chapter 23

LIFE AFTER TRANSPLANT

My life has changed so much since my transplant. I never waste a minute, and I value every day that I'm lucky enough to have. Every day is a bonus day as far as I am concerned. There's nothing I can't do in terms of living a normal life, and at the moment I'm just enjoying life and doing what I can to make the most of it. In May 2014, I went on a hot air balloon ride and tree trekking with my mom and brother Bill—things that were on my bucket list. In September 2014, Kyle, Sarah, my mom, and me took a trip to Disney World as a celebratory holiday for my having survived a year post-transplant.

My new liver has given me back my life in so many ways. Instead of sleeping *a lot*—at least twelve hours a day, and even more right before transplant—now I am able to stay awake the entire day. This is a new concept. I still get eight or nine hours of sleep each night, but now I don't need to nap every single day. That afternoon tiredness and lull in my energy level is no longer there. I figure I have gained at least three or four hours of awake time per day. I spend that extra time with my family. My kids are no longer propped in front of the TV watching a movie or playing video games while I sleep. I go for bike rides with them and play in the backyard. I bake cookies and make craft projects. My husband doesn't have to listen to me complain that I'm tired all the time; now he has to deal with me having more time to shop!

I'll have to be followed by the TGH Liver Transplant Clinic for the rest of my life. I don't mind, because I've developed a pleasant relationship with Dr. Renner and my nurse coordinator, Jill. At this point in time (March 2015), my appointment frequency has been reduced to yearly appointments. I was going to the clinic almost monthly, so this is a nice change. Now I don't have to fight Toronto traffic as often or pay expensive parking fees. My blood work frequency has also been reduced. Since I'm a year out, I still have to be poked and prodded at the lab, but only every three months. My veins are just barely holding up, so the fewer pokes, the better. I only have two good veins left, one in each arm. The rest of my veins are scarred from years of IVs and blood draws.

I had a few setbacks along the way, but with modern medicine and an excellent transplant team behind me, my condition eventually stabilized. My liver enzymes were elevated in February of this year, so Dr. Renner put me back on prednisone. My liver enzymes have stayed "perfect" for a few months now, so my current daily dose of prednisone has been reduced to only five milligrams. I hope to one day entirely and permanently cut off my relationship with prednisone, but since it's a relationship that started in 1987, when I was thirteen-years-old, I don't know if that will ever be the case.

When my liver enzymes increased in February, Dr. Renner could not, without my undergoing another liver biopsy, definitively determine whether I was experiencing a slight rejection or a possible return of my autoimmune hepatitis, since both elicit the same symptoms. My liver enzymes were only *slightly* elevated, so Dr. Renner didn't feel a liver biopsy was warranted at that time. I couldn't agree more! Eventually my liver enzymes returned to normal after a few of my medications were tweaked.

Dr. Renner and Jill told me that rejection does not mean I will lose my liver, but it is very important to begin treatment as soon as possible to avoid further complications. Rejection can usually be treated successfully with medication. Increasing the doses of anti-rejection medications, or adding or combining different anti-rejection medications, usually treats rejection. Although the risk of rejection decreases over time, it is always a possibility, and I will have to be concerned for the rest of my life about rejection or the return of my disease. Taking good care of myself, taking my medications as prescribed, and having my blood tests done regularly will help decrease my risk of rejection. Good communication with my transplant team and following my care routine are key factors for a successful outcome after transplant. I am willing to do whatever it takes to care for my new liver. After going through everything I just went through to be transplanted, I feel it is my duty to take good care of myself. I don't ever want to be re-transplanted—once is enough!

Not everything is perfect with my health. I wish it were, but I still have abnormal creatinine and hemoglobin. My slightly elevated creatinine means my kidney function is still a little off, and since kidney function and hemoglobin go hand in hand, my hemoglobin is lower than it should be (in the low 100s when it should be over 125). I can feel that my hemoglobin is low. I find I huff and puff a little more when doing exercise. Perhaps in time, my kidney function and hemoglobin will return to normal.

I make a conscious effort to drink more water to help me urinate more frequently and eliminate some of the excess creatinine from my body. I was told to drink two litres of fluid a day. After being fluid-restricted for so many years, it is difficult to do. But I purchased a BPA-free water bottle and keep track of my fluid intake. I drink mostly water and fruit juice and have eliminated caffeinated drinks and colas (which I seldom drank to begin with). I also follow a low-sodium diet and eat healthy, which is easy for me because I am a fruit lover and like raw vegetables, especially peas, beans, and carrots from our garden. I make meals and bake from scratch so I can control the ingredients and steer clear of additives like added salt and the mystery ingredients in prepared foods—things like *tartrazine*, *silicon dioxide*, and *disodium guanylate*—whatever those are? Sure, I indulge in comfort foods like potato chips or dark chocolate, but overall, I mind what I eat.

I asked my transplant coordinator for her thoughts on consuming alcohol. Jill told me that liver recipients are considered ambassadors of liver transplantation and should set a good example by avoiding alcohol. We should be respectful of our new livers—our gift of life. Plus, Jill said she can tell if patients are consuming alcohol because their AST and ALT liver enzymes often increase. Jill said that zero consumption is best, but that I could have a *tiny* amount of red wine or champagne—enough for a toast—at a wedding or special occasion. I told Jill that if I were never to have alcohol again that would be fine by me. I would rather have a healthy liver and live longer. Liver disease is too often associated with alcoholism, which is a shame because most people living with liver disease do not routinely consume alcohol. In fact, most of the recipients of liver transplants I know have never had a drink in their lives.

Transplant recipients have a lot on their plates. We have to take medications at specific times for the rest of our lives, attend numerous appointments, visit the lab frequently, be mindful of what we eat and drink, be in tune with any changes in our bodies suggestive of a rejection, and do our best to avoid germs. We are willing to do what it takes because we have been given a second chance at life, and we are grateful for that! But we don't live in a bubble despite being immunocompromised. We just make sure we steer clear of known illnesses and infection and wash our hands *a lot*. Knowing that an illness or infection can more easily make me sick and for a longer period of time, I have become a germaphobe, which makes life challenging when I live in a house with two little germ carriers.

No matter how often I harp on the kids to wash their hands and even squirt hand sanitizer on them, their dirty little germ-infested hands touch things that I touch. In April 2014, my husband and kids became afflicted with a short-lived gastrointestinal bug. Around

1 a.m. one night, Sarah peered into our room. The rancid smell woke us before she softly said, "I feel sick, Mommy and Daddy."

All nurses have a weakness, and vomit is mine. I quickly pulled a surgical mask out of the hallway closet and covered my mouth and nose. Then I did what any transplant mom would do—I ran to the basement to escape the germs. I left my husband to clean up Sarah, along with her pajamas, bedding, stuffed animals, and bedroom carpet.

Not long after, Kevin and Kyle came down with the bug as well. I was paranoid that I was going to get sick and be hospitalized. But I didn't get sick—shocking, I know. Maybe my immune system is getting stronger? It was likely my obsessive handwashing and avoidance of germs that kept me from catching this nasty bug. I carried a bottle of hand sanitizer in one pocket and my own hand towel in another for a couple of days. I designated the downstairs bathroom to myself and used bleach on all the faucets, light switches, and doorknobs, anywhere my sick family touched. I opened up the windows and aired out the house, hoping the germs would magically blow out the windows. Most importantly, I avoided my family. I couldn't hug my kids to make them better, or rub their backs to comfort them during their sickness like most moms. It was hard to watch them suffer and not be able to give them that snuggle they needed.

I was given a year off from work for surgical leave and wasn't expected to return until July 2014. Not only was I physically unable to do my job, but working in a hospital, where germs lurk everywhere, also puts my immunocompromised body at risk of acquiring an infection. I needed to develop my immune system again first. The transplant team told me I had the immune system of a baby and it would take time to build itself up. Avoiding the gastrointestinal illness that plagued my family proved I could protect myself from getting sick. *Handwashing, handwashing, handwashing—excessively!*

On March 25, eight months post-transplant, I retrieved my pink heart scrubs out of my bedroom closet, donned my stethoscope around my neck, and clipped on my name badge; it was time to re-enter the working world. I went back to work early because I was ready, and my transplant team agreed. I was assigned to a modified work schedule for a few weeks, then I was thrown into the deep end and worked three twelve-hour shifts in a row. I wasn't physically tired and didn't need to use the staff couch for naps during breaks. I had the physical energy to work twelve hours without crashing. The only thing I noticed was how sore my feet were. I was used to sitting and putting my feet up throughout the day. After twelve hours of running around our busy cardiac unit, my feet were throbbing and burning. When I got home after those initial twelve-hour shifts, Kyle offered to rub my feet for a small fee—one dollar for ten minutes. I took him up on the offer.

Returning to work made me feel normal again. I woke up with a purpose. Yes, I enjoyed sleeping in all those months and not having to wake to an alarm clock, but I was ready to be a nurse again. I enjoy being a nurse (most of the time!) and caring for others who are sick. Since returning to my full-time job as a cardiology nurse, I find I am now more empathetic toward patients. I don't feel I am a better nurse, because I like to think I was a good nurse in the first place. But I certainly feel I can relate to my patients on a more personal level.

A man who had a massive heart attack at his home was brought to the ER. He spent a week in the ICU, and once he was stable, he was transferred to our inpatient cardiology unit. I was the first nurse to care for him in our unit. He was heartbroken, literally and figuratively. He told me he is a single dad to a sixteen-year-old and, at fifty-one-years- old, a heart attack should never have happened. He felt bad that he didn't take good care of himself and heavily smoked and drank. I sat next to the patient on his bed and explained his angiogram results on a plastic heart model and helped him understand why he needed bypass surgery. After our teaching moment, I rested my hand on his forearm and told him, "You survived. You were given a second chance at life. There is a reason you are still here. Your son still has his father. Please take care of yourself, you have the power to make better choices in life." He cried and thanked me for giving him "a little pep talk." I never used to know what to say to patients after they experienced a life-threatening event. After nearly dying myself, I find it easier to know just the right thing to say to patients who need words of encouragement. He later showed me his "zipper" scar—he too survived surgery.

On admission to our unit, nurses ask patients if they are registered organ and tissue donors. I used to dread asking this question because I was afraid I would make patients think they were going to die during their hospitalization. Now, I always ask that question with confidence. Remarkably, many patients, and their family members, are registered. Some patients even whip out their OHIP card and proudly show off *Donor* inscribed on the back. I always thank them. When patients say they are not registered, I ask them if they would like to, and if they say yes, I help them through the process on the beadonor.ca website. It has been my mission to increase donor registration rates through my contact with patients and hospital staff. During my first week back on full regular duty, I registered six patients. Let's continue to get the word out there and increase those registration rates so that no one dies waiting for their life-saving organ.

Of course, I have the perfect job for increasing organ and tissue donation awareness. I included a paragraph in April's edition of our *Grapevine* in-house newsletter informing staff that April is organ and tissue donation awareness month and encouraging them to register their consent. I've passed around green organ-donation pens and ribbon pins. I have posted transplant stories and left a bag of green ribbon pins on our hallway bulletin board. My story was included in the April edition of St. Mary's newsletter, *Suture Line*. And, TGLN wrote a short story for Nursing Week in the May edition of *Hospital News*, a newspaper distributed in hospitals across Canada. I have shared my story and encouraged people to become registered donors during public speaking engagements. Speaking to a high school health class was one of my favourite teaching moments, as most of the class were sixteen-years-old—old enough to register their consent to donate.

I am proud of my story and want people to know that organ donation works. I am able to work full-time again. I never thought that would be possible. I get a lump in my throat and a warm, fuzzy feeling when co-workers come up to me and give me a hug and say things like, "You are amazing, you look really good," or, "Wow, you look healthy again, your colour is back, you look like you are feeling much better." My first weeks back at work weren't as overwhelming as I had anticipated. Sure, I had to remember things all over again, make sure I didn't make any errors, and keep up with the fast pace of our unit. But I received such a warm welcome back and much needed support from co-worker friends. They made the transition back to work a lot easier.

I do feel "normal" being back at work. For the most part my body is co-operating. My hands have a slight tremor at times, likely from the Prograf, so my fine motor skills aren't quite what they used to be. Opening medication packages and connecting IV lines can be a little difficult when my hands shake. Patients have noticed the mild tremors and often help open a package or remove a lid from a vial. I've had to learn to ask for help. Bending and twisting into certain positions, or boosting patients in bed, can elicit some incisional pain. I have to remind myself to be careful and not overdo it. I am particularly cautious about entering isolation rooms, and adamantly avoid those with patients who have confirmed cases of influenza, tuberculosis, E. coli, or C. difficile (two gastrointestinal-related infections). Acquiring one of these infections could be serious and land me back in the hospital.

During the first month back to work, I visited occupational health to check in and provide updates with how I was doing. I always told the staff, "I'm doing fine," because really, I was. I had no complaints or concerns. Everything was smooth sailing. Then on one of my shifts, my patient was scheduled for a permanent pacemaker. When a patient requires a pacemaker, a nurse must accompany that patient to the operating room because he or she is connected to a heart monitor. The OR doors were open, and I watched as staff counted instruments, adjusted the lighting, and moved a few tables around. The scene gave me a flashback; it looked like the transplant OR. The staff looked like the nurses who prepped me. The blue scrub cap covering my hair was the same. The smell of bleach, the brightness, and the shiny sterile instruments and tables—they were just like I remembered. I could feel my heart race. My palms became sweaty. I felt a little faint. Thankfully, the patient asked to use a urinal, which snapped my mind out of the moment—a much-needed distraction. I didn't expect this wave of emotion to take hold. I wiped away the tears before handing my patient his urinal.

Being back at work also allowed me to once again earn an income to help support our family. I received fifteen weeks of disability benefits through Employment Insurance from Service Canada, but after that time, I no longer qualified for additional benefits. Because I was part-time at St. Mary's Hospital at the time, I wasn't entitled to sick benefits. I had accrued extras costs for my medications and frequent trips to Toronto General Hospital, and had had to pay for medical supplies such as compression stockings and a walker. Kevin's extended medical plan helped us out, but we only had 80 percent coverage. During my surgical leave, co-worker friends from 3 East Inpatient Cardiology and 500 Medicine Unit (where I stayed as a patient) helped us out financially through fundraisers, for which I cannot thank them enough. Still, while we were a family of four living on one income, times were tight and we had to watch the budget closely.

To Kyle and Sarah, having a transplant is just something that is done to make people better. It's like sticking a Band-Aid on a cut, and *presto!* The cut is healed—no big deal! I think it is adorable to watch them play transplant. One time, Sarah was wrapped in blankets to keep her warm and had a magazine to read while she waited for the surgeon. Kyle, the surgeon, used my cooking tongs to remove

Sarah's organs for transplant, and then they used towels and Band-Aids to patch up Sarah. I'm not sure who got all of Sarah's organs, but I think I heard the kids pretend they were transplanting them into Sarah's stuffed animals and dolls. I'm sure they were put to good use. Another time, Kyle and Sarah found a large piece of cardboard in the garage. Kyle cut out a person the size of himself, and he and Sarah pretended their cardboard man was having a transplant. They cut out a liver, a heart, lungs, and a kidney. I told them they could also cut out a second kidney, a pancreas, and intestines. By the time they were done transplanting all the organs, the poor cardboard man had a big hole in his torso. Kyle told me, "Mommy, our cardboard man saved lots of people today."

If Band-Aids and towels were all I'd needed to help me, recovery would have been a cinch. This past year has had its ups and downs, but overall I can't complain. My incision is what it is: ugly (in my opinion), itchy (especially when I get sweaty), and tight. My whole abdomen feels tight and restricted. The tightness is worse after I sit too long in one position, and first thing in the morning after I wake up. The more I move, the more pliable the incision becomes. I have areas around the incision that are still numb, and that just feels weird—like those areas are not part of my body.

In a funny sort of way, I feel like I've gone through puberty again in the last year. Once all the fluid was drained out of my body, I went down to 110 pounds—*a sack of bones*. Then as time passed, I got my period. I developed breasts. My hips filled out. I blossomed into an adult-looking woman. My body regained its original shape and size, like memory foam. The only thing different about my body now is my battle scar—my peace-sign scar—proof I went through hell to survive. But I did survive, and made it to my fortieth birthday, one of my goals. A simple goal, really, but one I'd prayed I would make.

At nine months post-transplant, I started biking the five-kilometer route to and from work again. I was gardening and walking a lot, and I joined an exercise class at the community centre. My physical strength was improving, and I put it to the test. On April 26,

2014, my husband, kids, and I participated in the annual Waterloo Transplant Trot. Our intention was to have the kids scooter while we *leisurely walked* the five-kilometer through Waterloo Park, but about 1 km into the race, the scooter gang was nowhere in sight. We were afraid they'd gone off-course. A friend of Kyle's was with them who is known for disappearing. Kevin and I upped the pace and ran. Kevin was wearing loose jeans that kept falling down. I hadn't run in quite some time. We were quite the pair. We eventually caught up with the kids. Sarah wanted to continue scooting fast, so I ran alongside her. She was my cheering squad: "Go, Mommy, we are almost there . . . I see another green arrow, go, Mommy." I ran most of the way, and when I needed short breaks, I walked *really* fast. To my surprise, my Life Donation Awareness Association friends were at the finish line and announced that I was the first transplant recipient to finish. "I don't run," I told them. Really I don't. I *used* to run, but not anymore. If it weren't for Sarah encouraging me on her scooter, I would never have run. I guess I still have it in me. But I must admit, my body paid for it later that day, and for two days afterwards—it hurt to even get out of bed.

During my night-time prayers, I always thank my donor and donor family for saving my life. A near-death experience has changed my life. Many people who have been on the brink of death will tell you they look at life in a new light and appreciate the little things much more. I give my children tighter hugs, and we hug more often. I do more things with my family and appreciate my children more. They are one of the reasons I am thankful to still be alive.

I am also thankful that my husband and I could celebrate our fourteenth anniversary in August 2014. I just have to say what a wonderful husband I have! He saw me at my absolute worst in the weeks before surgery and immediately after surgery. I know I didn't look or behave like the person he married. It isn't easy to have a conversation with your thirty-nine-year-old spouse about her *wishes*, just in case a liver doesn't become available in time.

I see beauty now in the smallest things—flowers in full bloom, cocooning butterflies, the exact blue colour of the sky. I realized that there is no promise of tomorrow. You are given such a short time, and you never know when your time will run out. Mine was almost up a year ago. It may be hard to truly appreciate this if you've never had to think about death, but I understand now how important it is to treasure your life, to make it worthwhile. Spend your life doing things that make you happy, because you may not have the chance later. My life has become fuller, more beautiful, and more full of gratitude. It's funny how laid back I have become. I don't sweat the small stuff anymore. Why be in a hurry to get things done? If the beds aren't made today, does it really matter? Life is too short and too precious to allow it to fly by. Stop and smell the roses—I certainly did the last time I was in Belleville and wandered through the Corby Rose Garden. They smell fantastic.

I am just about two years post-transplant now—two more years I was able to live because of my donor and his or her family. Two more years of life because of the support and wonderful care provided by my transplant team. Two more years to spend with my family and friends. My first "liverversary" was celebrated on my daughter's seventh birthday. She and I celebrated together. I didn't have a liver-shaped cake (Sarah vetoed the idea). I celebrated one year with my new liver by being able to enjoy and take part in my daughter's birthday party. Being able to wrap my arms around my blonde-haired princess and see her turn seven was the best post-transplant present ever. Life does go on, and I'm still in the game.

Chapter 24

RAISING AWARENESS:
OTHERS' TRANSPLANT JOURNEYS

F our months after my transplant, I joined the Life Donation Awareness Association (LDAA) as another way to "pay it forward" and meet other people with recycled body parts. LDAA is a collaboration of pre- and post-transplant recipients, family, and friends; donor family members; and other community volunteers who build awareness and support for organ and tissue donation. There are four chapters of LDAA across southern Ontario. I belong to is the Midwest chapter—the region of Waterloo and surrounding townships. Our mission is to raise public awareness of organ and tissue donation and to encourage conversations and family discussions about, and registration and consent for, organ and tissue donation, community by community. We want to touch people with our stories, dispel misconceptions, and share the reality of life before and after transplant. Some members have been kind enough to share with me, and have given me permission to share with you, their heartfelt stories.

When LDAA members speak at a public engagement or have a booth at a community event, the public is able to put a face to organ and tissue donation. I am still amazed whenever someone comes up to me and says, "You are young . . . I thought transplant recipients were old." Most of us organ recipients are young (if you think forty-one is young). Or, people will say, "You look so healthy . . . would never have guessed you received a new liver." I feel our group shows the public that yes, recipients are healthy and active individuals—that organ donation really works.

It is a reality that someone in Canada dies every three days waiting for an organ transplant. I saw those people in hospital. They were sick and lying in their hospital beds, waiting to be given a second chance at life. Some patients were fortunate and received their gift of life. But many didn't survive because an organ wasn't available to save them in time—they had to wait too long. I can't begin to tell you how sickening it was to listen to patients suffer while waiting. Uncomfortable moaning by dying patients echoed throughout the unit. I heard a young woman in her twenties plead with her nurse, "Please make this hurt stop, please." Alarms sounded when patients' heart rates dipped too low because their hearts were failing. The oxygen monitors beeped nonstop when their lungs weren't providing enough oxygen. Liver patients were yellow and swollen, often confined to their beds. It was devastating to listen to families painfully wail in heartache as they said goodbye to their loved ones because an organ wasn't available in time to save them. A man waiting for a kidney, who I often visited with in the TV lounge, told me, "I am not ready to die yet." His eyes welled up in tears as he told me, "I have young kids and a wife. They need me. I don't want my boys to grow up without a dad."

Like so many thankful recipients, I want more than anything for no one to die waiting for an organ transplant. In Ontario, over 1,500 people are presently wait-listed. No progress can be attained without action from the donor community. One organ donor can save up to eight lives, and one tissue donor can enhance as many as seventy-five more. Each of us has the incredible power to create change; each of us carries the gift of life!

When donor family members speak at organ and tissue donation awareness engagements, the audience listens with Kleenex in hand. Donor family members can not only touch the hearts of listeners but also answer questions and educate the public regarding the actual donation. The first time I heard Janine speak about her dad, the man she looked up to and the person who helped guide her through many years of her life, I cried (along with just about everyone else in the crowd). I cried because it was difficult to hear how sad it is to lose someone so close, yet be faced with the decision to donate—a decision that has to be made in a time of heartache and sorrow. I was reminded, as I am every day, of my gratitude toward my donor and donor family.

Janine's story gave me some insight into the organ donation process from the perspective of the donor family. Janine's father passed away on November 11, 2009, from cerebral amyloid angiopathy (congophilic angiopathy), a spontaneous brain bleed that was likely the result of a genetic predisposition in combination with uncontrolled blood pressure issues. Her dad was only sixty-four-years-old.

JANINE'S STORY

I have a medical background, so I knew that we were in a "bad place" before they actually told any of us outright. I recall discussing the idea of organ donation with my brother while travelling from Cambridge Memorial Hospital to Hamilton General Hospital. I just had a feeling that was where we were heading.

We had an official update meeting with my dad's neurologist and his bedside nurses on the Monday morning following a weekend filled with extensive testing. During the meeting we were told he was "vegetative," meaning that he had less than 10 percent brain function. However, because he still technically had a small amount of brain function, he was not considered "brain dead" at that time.

We were given several options during the meeting. One of those options was to speak with the Trillium Gift of Life Network (TGLN) team to decide if we would like to consider organ donation. Our decision to donate or not to donate would directly affect the path the medical team took as far as my dad's "treatment" went. In our case, we would have to decide (at that time) if we wanted to remove my dad from all of the machines first. Doing so would subsequently allow him to pass from a cardiac death because, again, technically, he still had minimal brain function.

We met with someone from TGLN the next day. We were all in a small "family room" for about an hour. The questions were primarily about my dad's health and medical history. We were also asked about my dad's sexual history, his family history, and a little bit about his travel and work history and any possible exposure to infectious material or diseases. Basically the primary screening conversation was to see if there was anything that would have sent out a red flag and rendered him unable to donate before more extensive testing was started. The TGLN coordinator explained the specific testing procedures.

The coordinator also explained the process of organ donation in extensive medical terms to me, and in "regular" terms to my brother and other family members. The assessment of each organ's viability would happen after we removed my dad from life support, after he was pronounced deceased. The cause of death would be that his heart stopped beating. How long it would take for his heart to stop was an unknown; some people pass quickly, others hang on for days. After two hours, the organs become less viable and donation is not always possible. Skin and/or tissue donation could still be an option depending on several other technicalities post–cardiac death. The TGLN coordinator was very specific in explaining the difference between "brain death" and what was happening with my dad at that moment. Although I understood everything, it was helpful to have a third party explain all of the information to my brother and our extended family.

As it turned out, my dad slipped into full brain death on Wednesday. Removing him from the machines was then *not* an option if we still wished to donate his organs. Because the doctors had now pronounced him brain dead, the very machines we were supposed to remove were now what were keeping the organs viable.

Upon further testing post-death, it was determined that my dad's heart and lungs had suffered too much damage to be used for transplant purposes. My dad's eyes were not that great on a good day, so it was decided that they were also unsuitable for transplant, but they were sent to the Eye Institute to be used for specific research purposes.

The thing that struck me at the time, and even now, was how completely respectful the staff were toward my dad while all of this was happening. They spoke to him like he could hear them, and someone stayed with him from the moment we consented to move forward with the donation analysis on Tuesday until the moment he passed away. More important, and what I'm most grateful for, is the fact that the same TGLN coordinator stayed with my dad throughout the surgical process; while the organs were harvested until he was taken to the mortuary. It was very comforting knowing he was so well taken care of during his final moments.

———

My friend, and heart recipient, Andrea Clegg founded the LDAA Midwest chapter in 2010. I asked Andrea how the group was started.

> "There was a lot of organizing, correspondence, and media efforts prior to the first meeting, to gain contacts and members. I connected with an individual who had started a group in a different area and picked her brain for advice. I connected with the local TGLN organ and tissue donation coordinator because she had previously organized

volunteer events at the local hospital and encouraged more efforts in our area. She provided me with all of the important information about organ and tissue donation to properly pass it on. I was friends with others waiting on an artificial heart (LVAD) and they supported the initiative. Basically, I just called a bunch of people together using media stories and the contacts from TGLN. We had eighteen people attend the first meeting—most are still members. Everyone was very encouraged. Some people had experience with organ and tissue donation events and speaking, so that helped get LDAA off the ground. We utilized connections to community service groups, organizations, workplaces, and schools to just get out there. I can't say I had "all my ducks in a row" for the first meeting, but somehow we all generated a relationship and began to grow. It's funny to look back.

"The Life Donation Awareness Association is a very active and successful awareness group. I am proud to say that the individuals who have joined together to raise awareness for organ and tissue donation in our community have contributed to the increase in registration by about 5 percent over the past couple years! With the addition of beadonor.ca and media pushes from TGLN, we have grabbed on to the attention and have been a part of many events throughout the community. My measure of success comes when I visit a random place with my organ donation paraphernalia and someone says, out of nowhere, 'I just registered!' Or, 'I heard a speaker about organ donation just a little while ago!' What a great moment. We are making an impact."

I knew of Andrea long before we actually met. She was a patient at St. Mary's Hospital in the inpatient cardiology unit where I work. I wasn't working at St. Mary's yet when Andrea was a patient there, but I knew of her story from my co-workers. How many newlyweds spend their honeymoon in a hospital? Her story was the talk of the hospital and a featured story in local newspapers, on Global News' *16x9* TV program, and on the TGLN and beadonor.ca websites. My kids think of her as a celebrity.

Andrea and her remarkable transplant journey have certainly inspired and motivated me and many others. Her story demonstrates something I sincerely believe, "that it's in your weakest moments you find your true strength."

ANDREA'S STORY

In spring 2008, strange symptoms started occurring with my health. I felt extra tired at my exercise classes and had incidents of increased heart rates. I went to see my family doctor several times. It was thought that my birth control pill was creating side effects, so I immediately stopped taking it. We also had discussions of possible strokes, as they can be a side effect of the pill. When I had a strange shock down my left side, I immediately went to the nearest emergency room. They did a CT scan, set me up for a neurology follow-up, and sent me on my way.

The weekend of May 10, 2008, I felt really awful. I couldn't walk my dogs and did not want to do anything. That Sunday, my mom took me to the emergency clinic and was prepared to fight to get them to figure out what was going on. She wheeled me into the hospital with a wheelchair. My resting heart rate was over 130 beats per minute. They finally did an echo (ultrasound of the heart) and ECG and told me that I had dilated cardiomyopathy. I felt relieved at this point to know what was happening. Little did I know what the future would hold.

Dilated cardiomyopathy occurs when the left ventricle, the heart's main pumping chamber, doesn't pump as efficiently as a healthy heart's. The muscles of the left ventricle stretch and become thinner (dilate). Dilation causes the heart muscle to weaken, and over time, the condition can cause heart failure. Often, the cause of dilated cardiomyopathy can't be determined.

I had been with Shaun for about four years prior to my diagnosis. We'd bought a house together, adopted some pets, and discussed our future. Three weeks after I was diagnosed with heart disease, he proposed to me. The future in general had become unclear, but we knew one thing for sure: however long we had, we wanted to spend that time together. He is my rock, my knight in shining armour. He has made this disease easier to cope with and has given me something to fight for. At the time, I didn't understand what that really meant and how true it would become.

I was told that I would just have to live with 10 to 20 percent left-sided heart function. I was not severe enough to be added to the transplant list, although I was being followed at an outpatient clinic. Three months after diagnosis, the doctors decided to implant a defibrillator (ICD), affectionately named Ivan, to control arrhythmias and prevent sudden death—a blunt comfort. The ICD is implanted under the skin along the right upper chest and is designed to give a shock if it detects a life-threatening cardiac arrhythmia.

I wasn't in a condition to work as of yet, so I made wedding planning my job. I planned it all. It was so much fun. I made my flowers, the cake, the wedding favours, the invitations, and the thank-you cards, and organized everything. We married in May of 2009 and the day was absolutely beautiful. I married the man of my dreams, committing my life to him in front of all my dearest family and friends. As the night passed on, we had dinner and began our speeches. Well, Ivan was not happy with the speech and decided to make his presence known. Two minutes into our speech, my heart rate increased to an unsafe rate and Ivan fired three times. My new husband caught me before I fell to the floor.

As I understand it, my heart rate was over 180 beats per minute for two minutes, which was too high a rate for a sick heart and triggered the ICD. The first time it fired, my heart went into ventricular tachycardia; the second and third times, it did not control the arrhythmia. It was actually after the third shock that I got myself out of the dangerous rhythm with the help of a nurse at my side. The paramedics took me, in my wedding gown, to St. Mary's Hospital.

I was taken to the ER, so the nurses and staff planned a little party for us in the hospital that night. We were able to cut the cake, throw the bouquet to single nurses, and have a toast. They treated me wonderfully and made the difficult experience a little better.

It was after the wedding that my condition declined significantly. The failing left side of my heart also caused the right side to fail. Other organs were being affected as well. After spending two weeks in St. Mary's at the beginning of October 2009, the doctors started talking transplant. I spent four days at Toronto General Hospital for testing to be placed on the transplant list. Testing typically takes four *months*, so things moved fast. I remember when the nurse came in to tell me that I was approved for a new heart. I try my best to be strong at all times, but that moment went straight to my heart, literally. On October 22, 2009, I was listed. It gave me a feeling of hope and strength—hope that I would do the things I loved to do again, and strength that I could push through whatever came next. I was aware of the risks but was convinced that I would succeed.

After I was listed, I experienced the fight of my life. Hooked up to about fifteen IVs did nothing to improve my condition. I had waited three days for a heart to become available and would not be able to wait another day without help. I stopped eating, drinking, sitting up, even sleeping. The echo showed that my heart had stopped moving.

On October 25, the doctors implanted a Left Ventricular Assist Device (LVAD), also known as an artificial heart, to pump blood through my body, since my heart was no longer able to do it alone. This was life-saving surgery, and I feel it was my second chance at life. Its purpose is a "bridge to transplant." The LVAD connects to the base of the left side of the heart and also to the aortic valve. The blood is detoured this way and then circulated through the body. The pump isn't really a pump, but provides a continuous blood flow. I hardly had a pulse or blood pressure. It was difficult to read vitals on me, but the doctors knew what to look for and monitored me very carefully.

At first, the LVAD hurt like words I cannot type here. I am smaller than the average patient and the LVAD barely fit. For a good three months or so I was in constant pain. The LVAD would rub against my ribs, and I would feel its ten-pound weight shift whenever I moved. I also had pain associated with having had open-heart surgery and had to take painkillers.

I could feel the LVAD humming if I put my hand over it or when I didn't have a shirt on. I was battery powered. The battery would last about fifteen hours. Then the LVAD was plugged into the wall for recharging. There was also a backup battery just in case.

There are some limitations for a person being supported by an LVAD. I had to avoid any significant static shock, such as vacuuming or touching TV screens. I could not swim or be immersed in any water. I had a shower bag that was particularly designed for the LVAD. I could not jump, since the LVAD could disconnect from my heart. I could not be in a car seat that had airbags because if they were to go off, they could disconnect the pump. I could not lie or sleep on my stomach because of the drive-line exit site. It seems like a lot, but really I just got used to not doing particular things.

I waited fourteen months for my heart. The wait was not terrible for me because I lived on the LVAD. During my wait, I had one false call in April 2010. I was sleeping soundly after a big night at my parents' house in Niagara Falls. It was only the second night in six months that we were away from home. I was dreaming that I was with nurses I knew from volunteering earlier in the week, and they were getting a call with a ringtone I didn't recognize. I woke myself up, and then it hit me what the sound was. It was my pager to notify me of a possible available heart. I called the number left on my pager and it was for . . . another pager. *Seriously?* They called back right away, but it felt like the longest thirty seconds ever. The lady was very friendly and calm and told me that they think they have a heart for me. She gave me instructions of where to go and what to expect. She told me to take my morning pills with a glass of water because sometimes "things happen" and it might not be right for me.

Not long after we got to the hospital, the surgeon came in to see us. It was Dr. Cuisimano. He had done my LVAD surgery. He told me that they might remove Ivan the ICD, since patients typically don't need an ICD after having a transplant. Even though Ivan and I had been through a lot together, we were both okay to retire our relationship. Shaun and I were also briefly informed of the risks involved in the surgery, which we were partly aware of already. We were told that it wouldn't be unlikely for the surgery to run six or eight hours. I didn't mind, but that's a long time for the family to wait.

Dr. Cuisimano told us that he was going himself to see the donor heart because it was in town. He said we would know in a couple of hours if it was good enough for me—it's hard to tell if a heart is in good condition until a surgeon has it in his hands to evaluate.

After a couple of hours, another of the surgeons came in to tell us that the heart was not good enough. They wanted the best heart to give me the best chance. They found some signs of coronary artery disease, or something like that, in the donor heart. I could tell that this was news the doctors did not want to share, but while it was disappointing, I didn't feel too bummed because I knew that it was in my best interest—*just a dress rehearsal.*

I received a transplant on December 21, 2010. It truly saved my life. If a transplant had not been an option, I would not be alive to share my story. I am able to plan for the future. I am a contributing member of society. I have continued on the path where I left off, with much more in my life. It's been a long road, but I feel I have found the right direction and, along with it, where I can make a mark on this world. I have a thankful heart and value for life. I have new friends, new experiences, and passion for connecting with other people who have faced challenges similar to mine.

I sent my donor family a thank-you letter, and regardless of whether they choose to respond, I respect and appreciate them all the same. I want to say thank you to them and to all donor families. It is with your selfless giving at your most difficult moment that many people have their lives back. As a recipient, I feel your loss and grieve for your loved one, even though I never knew him or her. You have saved my family from enduring the same loss of their wife, daughter, sister, and friend. I hope you find peace in knowing the many lives your kindness has touched.

—

Joanna, Ryley's mom, is an active LDAA member. I met Joanna at the first LDAA meeting I attended. Her warm and welcoming demeanour made me feel instantly a part of the LDAA group. I must admit, I was a little nervous being the newbie and not knowing a single soul, but Joanna let me sit next to her as she typed meeting minutes.

I would like to share Ryley's story for a couple of reasons. First, Ryley is truly an amazing young girl who has experienced things in her short life that most people will never experience in their lifetime. Knowing that she is such a strong little girl, and is able to deal with all the poking and prodding in hospital, has made me realize that I shouldn't be such a wimp when it comes to needles. If a brave little girl like Ryley can do it, then I too can be brave.

Second, Ryley's story looks at organ transplantation from a parent's perspective. Ryley was a baby when she received her new heart and has no recollection of being sick and recovering from surgery. It was her parents who had to entrust Ryley's health and well-being to the hospital staff at The Hospital for Sick Children (SickKids), and who had the stress and worry to bear, along with a myriad of other emotions, I'm sure. I can't begin to imagine how many tears and sleepless nights they withstood.

I first met Ryley on a parade float at the Cambridge Santa Claus parade in 2013. She was holding a sign that read, in green and red letters, *I had a heart transplant 2006.* My daughter and I were on the float as well, with my *Liver recipient, July 21, 2013* sign decorated in Christmas lights and tinsel. When my children first met Ryley, they were surprised to learn that a child their age could receive an organ transplant.

RYLEY'S STORY— AS TOLD BY HER MOM, JOANNA

Our beautiful daughter Ryley was born on Father's Day in 2005, the best present a dad could ever get! Her birth was much anticipated, as we had been trying to start our family for the past five years, with some difficulty. There were no complications through the pregnancy and birth, and our daughter seemed to be healthy and happy. We attended all doctor's visits, and the public health nurse saw her a few times. Nobody knew just by looking at her that she was slowly dying.

When Ryley was two and a half months old, she had some episodes of vomiting and her breathing seemed laboured. After a few days of this, my mother's instinct said she needed to be seen by a doctor right away and we headed to a local walk-in clinic. The clinic was booked up for the night, so we made the decision to go to our local emergency room. We said if it weren't busy we would go in, but if it were busy, we would call our own doctor in the morning. Fate would have it that the waiting room of the emergency room was empty. Looking back, I think that may have saved Ryley's life.

As first-time parents, we expected that we were overreacting and would be told that she just had a bit of a "bug" and sent home.

Instead, our local doctor checked her over and sent her for a chest X-ray, and we soon found ourselves in an ambulance on our way to the Children's Hospital in London for more tests

When we arrived in London, doctors and nurses, trying to examine her and get blood, swarmed our tiny baby. Through all the commotion, I remember seeing the one doctor standing in the background, holding up the chest X-ray that had been done in our local hospital and saying, "enlarged heart." I didn't really know what that meant, but I knew it was bad. Soon a cardiologist came, the room emptied out, and he did an echo on Ryley. Within an hour of arriving, we had the diagnosis of dilated cardiomyopathy, or an enlarged heart. When the heart becomes enlarged and cannot effectively pump blood to the rest of your body, your other organs start to fill with fluid and shut down. With the severity of Ryley's enlargement, it was a miracle she was still alive. I asked the doctor if this meant she was going to die. He said no, but she would likely be a candidate for a heart transplant.

Ryley was given many medications, some put through an IV that was in her scalp because it was the only place they could find a vein in her tiny body. The doctors hoped these medications would lessen the load on her heart and it would heal. I remember another cardiologist doing another echo on her and just sitting there shaking his head. I was so numb.

With the severity of Ryley's heart failure, the only treatment option was a heart transplant. The closest pediatric heart transplant centre was SickKids in Toronto. She was to be transferred by helicopter there. Because of the weight restrictions in the helicopter, we were unable to accompany Ryley and would have to drive to Toronto to meet her. Seeing our little baby girl fly away from us was one of the hardest things we went through. I walked away from the helicopter bawling my eyes out. We did not know if she would still be alive by the time we got there.

Ryley did arrive at SickKids safely. Over the next few days, they were able to stabilize her on numerous cardiac medications, and after a week we were able to take her home. She remained at home for the next five months, with weekly visits to the hospital to monitor her condition, round-the-clock medication, and daily visits from a home care nurse. We watched and waited, hoping for a miracle recovery. But miracles sometimes come in ways we least expect them

We celebrated Ryley's first Christmas at home, but when we look back at the pictures, we can see she was really not well. In January 2006, Ryley's condition was getting worse. She was no longer putting on weight and she was vomiting more and more. Ryley was admitted to Children's Hospital in London on January 11, 2006, because of laboured breathing. On January 15, we sat down with the same cardiologist who had diagnosed her, and he gave us a choice. We could list her for transplant or take the route of palliative care—making her comfortable until she passed. We decided that it was time to list her for a heart transplant because we were not willing to let her go.

We were transferred that day back to SickKids in Toronto, where the assessment of whether Ryley was suitable to receive a heart began. On January 19, she received a feeding tube to help her get nutrition, as she no longer had the energy to eat, and she was officially listed for transplant.

After spending ten days in the Critical Care Unit (CCU), we received the call that they thought they had a heart for Ryley! Because Ryley was under a year old and her immune system had not developed, she was able to accept a heart that was not the same blood type as her own and not reject it. On January 29, Ryley received her gift of life—a new heart—and we received our miracle!

Ryley's surgery lasted five hours, and we were able to see her in CCU that evening. She remained in CCU only two days before being transferred back to the cardiac ward. Amazingly, only eleven days later, she was discharged from the hospital. The little baby who seemed so sad before had the biggest smiles now. How good her body must have felt to have a strong, working heart! We have called her Smyley Ryley ever since.

Transplant life is not perfect. Ryley takes medications that are hard on her body, and she has many tests to monitor her health. One day, she will need another transplant. But she is alive, she has an excellent quality of life, and you would never know all that she has gone through unless we told you. The only reason this is possible is because of her donor and his family. She would not be here today if the donor family had not made such a hard decision during one of the most tragic times of their lives, losing their own child. We are forever grateful to them.

Although we will not meet Ryley's donor family due to privacy laws, we are able to thank them in anonymous letters sent through our organ donation agency. We wrote letters to them three months after her transplant, and five years after. Around Ryley's seven-year anniversary, we received a letter back from her donor family. It must have been so hard for them to be able to put those words on paper, and we are so appreciative to them for letting us know they have received our letters. I hope they will always know how thankful we are for the gift of life they gave to our daughter. As a mother, I can only hope that knowing their son's heart is living on in our daughter brings them a small measure of comfort.

By registering to be an organ donor and discussing your wishes with your family, you can truly be a hero by saving the lives of up to eight recipients like Ryley after you are gone, and bringing joy to the lives of those who love them.

———

Living donation is an incredible expression of altruism and generosity. My friend Kelly, a liver recipient I met through LDAA, received her life-saving liver transplant through living organ donation. In 2011, the year Kelly was transplanted, 428 adult liver transplants were performed in Canada. Of those 428 liver transplants, forty-nine were from living donors. With his selfless gift, Kelly's uncle was one of those forty-nine.

KELLY'S STORY

My journey to transplant began when I was twenty-three-years-old and pregnant with my first child. My skin became very itchy, to the point where I was scratching it bloody. My family doctor dismissed it and told me that pregnant skin is itchy. Desperate for relief, I went to a dermatologist, who ordered blood work only to find that my liver enzymes were ten times as high as they should have been. The hope was that once I delivered the baby, everything would go back to normal. But this was not the case, and by then I was under the care of a new family doctor, who referred me to a hepatologist. My original diagnosis was primary biliary cirrhosis, which was later changed to primary sclerosing cholangitis.

My main symptoms were itchiness and fatigue. The itching kept me from sleeping at night, and I began sleeping all day instead, which made regular life extremely difficult. Imagine nine years of being covered in the worst rash of your life—only there is no rash—and being sleep-deprived the whole time. And try explaining to people that you are sick, when there is nothing to see! Over the years, people thought that it was helpful to say "stop scratching." *Gee, why didn't I think of that?* The itch was so exhausting and frustrating that it brought me to tears on many occasions. I tried every lotion, potion, and antidote to make it go away, but nothing worked. I resorted to sleeping with ice packs directly on my skin. During that time, I went on to have another child (with another torturous pregnancy) and continued to work full-time. I was fortunate to be able to work right up until my transplant. My biggest concern was that post-transplant, I would still itch out of habit. Part of me wasn't convinced that it wasn't all in my head.

I was listed November 5, 2010, after waiting nine years to become "sick enough" to need a transplant. Once I was listed, the process of identifying a live donor began. Potential donors fill out a sort of application and fax it to Toronto General Hospital. Candidates are tested in the order that the applications are received. By December, my younger brother had been tested and identified as a match, but he was refused due to his profession. At the time, he was a professional baseball player, and it was felt that the surgery could negatively impact his career. They went on to the next candidate, my uncle Ken (who was fifty-eight at the time). Testing on Ken was completed in early 2011, and our surgeries were scheduled for March second of that year.

Our surgeries were separate. My uncle went into the operating room first. The surgical team opens up the donor first to ensure that everything is as expected from the work-up and imaging that was done. Once that was confirmed, the surgical team called for me. Our surgeries were done in separate operating rooms, by separate surgical teams so that each of our best interests was top of mind.

I received my uncle's right lobe (the larger lobe). When I woke up, I felt immediately better. My itchiness was gone and I was able to get up, and was moving by the next day. Uncle Ken's recovery was a bit slower. Whereas I was ready to do laps around the step down unit, his body was recovering from a loss and he experienced pain and nausea. Ultimately, however, he was the first to leave the hospital. He left five days post-surgery, but I was there for ten days. I was definitely ready to leave on day five, but blood work and a biopsy showed rejection, so I spent five more days in hospital so that they could treat me with a heavy-duty steroid called Solu-Medrol. It only took eight weeks for each of our livers to grow back completely— how remarkable!

My liver transplant has changed me very much. All drug side effects aside, I am much more sensitive and emotional. I don't sweat the small stuff and find joy in the simple things in life. It's a gift of perspective, really. Most people spend their whole lives without it, until they are faced with adversity. It's a real blessing to get that perspective early in life so that it can be shared, and capitalized on. This life is not for taking for granted, and I intend to make the most out of it, personally and professionally. You are a changed person when you know people who are truly happy just to be alive and breathing. I definitely have a sense of obligation to pay it forward.

On March 2, 2015, I celebrated my fourth "liverversary." There are no words to express my gratitude to my uncle Ken for his selflessness and generosity. I have a wonderful life—two beautiful, healthy little boys, the unconditional love and support of family and friends, and a career that I am proud of. I can't wait to see where this road in life takes me and to see all of the things I can accomplish. I hope my uncle will be proud of the choices I make and the role model I will be. The most wonderful part of having a living donor is that I have the ability to tell him "thank you" whenever I want to. Without him, I wouldn't have this opportunity to build memories and have this amazing life.

Since my transplant, I have had the opportunity to participate in the World Transplant Games in Durban, South Africa, in the summer of 2013, and the Canadian Transplant Games in Moncton, New Brunswick, in the summer 2014. The games are incredible—being surrounded by hundreds of people who have received the gift of life through organ donation is really overwhelming and emotional. They are truly a living testament that organ donation works!

—

Shelly was my second roommate on the seventh floor transplant unit at TGH. She had survived her ordeal in the ICU and step down units and was recovering when we met. I had not had my transplant yet when we were roommates, so I bombarded Shelly with many questions: Does it hurt? How long was surgery? What's the ICU like? How are you held together, with staples? Shelly was in a lot of pain and felt really sick during recovery in hospital. I frequently heard her ask her nurse for pain medications. I felt bad that her pain kept her up at night. She also had a lot of swelling and extra fluid, so she was given a diuretic, which meant we had to compete for the bathroom.

Shelly was literally by my side, in the adjacent bed, when I was told the first liver was a no-go. She was also present when the transplant team delivered the awesome news the morning of July 21—the news that the second liver, my new liver, was transplantable. She shared in tears and prayers with me that life-changing weekend. She gave me a hug goodbye when I was on the gurney, ready to be wheeled to the operating room, which was especially comforting because my family could not be there. Shelly and I still stay in touch through email, and we have met each other once in the waiting room during early-morning clinic appointments on the twelfth floor of TGH. It is inspiring and comforting to know that she is doing so well post-transplant. And thanks to her gift of life, she was able to become a grandma in January 2014.

SHELLY'S STORY

I have lived with kidney disease and have been subjected to hospitals all my life. Like me, my grandmother, mother, and younger sister were all kidney dialysis patients. We have a familial disease called polycystic kidney disease (PKD). PKD is a genetic disorder characterized by the growth of numerous cysts in the kidneys. When cysts form in the kidneys, they are filled with fluid. PKD cysts can profoundly enlarge the kidneys while replacing much of the normal structure, resulting in reduced function and leading to kidney failure. My grandmother was not able to have a transplant, but my sister received her kidney in 2007, and my mother received hers in 2010. My mother and I each had a deceased donor, and my sister had a living donor, a close friend. It was a miracle that all three of us were able to receive a new life through transplants.

In addition to meeting other criteria such as blood typing and tests for viruses, potential recipients cannot be placed on a transplant list until they meet the requirement of waiting for five to seven years. Once I was officially listed in September 2012, I waited eleven months for my new kidney.

Prior to my transplant, I was on dialysis. I was also treated for high blood pressure and told to watch my diet. I had to limit the amount of sodium, potassium, and phosphorus in my diet. Basically I had to eat healthy and get a lot of exercise and rest. I followed these instructions, but unfortunately, I had to start peritoneal dialysis at home. A trial of peritoneal dialysis didn't work completely, and I had to go to the next stage of dialysis—home hemodialysis. Then I received the news that my creatinine levels were extremely high and I needed to go on hemodialysis at the hospital, where I could be watched more closely. It was nothing I was doing wrong; the disease was taking its course, and I was nearing total kidney failure. During my dialysis I was attending clinics and appointments at Toronto General Hospital, getting prepared for a transplant.

My husband and I had just started holidays and we were at our trailer in Madoc, Ontario, when our cell phone went off at 3:50 a.m. My husband answered it, but the signal was weak and we were disconnected. We called back only to be disconnected again. We realized it was someone from TGLN, and on our third call attempt we received the news that a kidney was available. We immediately left and headed to Toronto. There, they told me that I was the primary candidate. I was thrilled but was not sure at the time if the kidney was a match—we had to wait for blood test results to come back. We never called any family until we knew for sure. At around 2 p.m., the surgeon came in and said everything was good and I would be prepared for surgery, which was scheduled for 4 p.m. The only thing I remember after that is waking up around 1 a.m., and my husband smiling when I said, "Everything is good. My new kidney is working great and I am going to be all right."

My gift of life was given to me on July 15, 2013. I do not know who the donor was. I was told that it was a male, approximately nineteen-years-old, and he had been killed in a motor vehicle accident.

As a kidney recipient, I have a completely new outlook on life. I have been given a second chance by someone else's generosity and selflessness. I don't have to attend dialysis three times per week. I'm able to spend more time with my family, I have a lot more energy, and I feel truly blessed. I never take anything for granted. Words cannot express what I feel in my heart. The transplant team asks you to give your new organ a name. I named my new kidney "Grace" because by the grace of God I was able to receive this wonderful gift. I did write a letter to the donor's family expressing how sorry I was for their loss. I wanted them to know that because of their family member's generosity and giving, he is still living on in me. There isn't a day that goes by that I don't think about what I have received. I just wish that every person waiting for a transplant could receive a lifesaving gift.

—

It just so happens that there is another transplant recipient living on our quiet crescent in Kitchener—two recipients on one street, what are the chances? For Phil, what began in February 2006 as concern that a persistent bad cough would keep him from being allowed to be present at the birth of his first child, resulted in a diagnosis of dilated cardiomyopathy and ultimately, in September of that year, a heart transplant.

Phil and Andrea are our neighbours and our friends. Our kids are all around the same age and are friends as well, and attend the same public school. Phil and Andrea helped us out tremendously by looking after Kyle and Sarah when Kevin visited me in the hospital.

Phil and Andrea have been down the transplant road and understood the difficult journey we faced. When we had questions, they were our go-to friends for answers. I found the changes in my sense of taste bizarre, but was reassured to know that Phil's sense of taste had changed as well. I slept a lot those first few months at home, and it was calming to know that Phil slept just as much during his recovery. Phil and I can swap war stories and talk about crude things like incisions and bowel habits—things non-transplant people don't generally think of talking about.

Since I can see Phil and Andrea's house from our house, I can be a nosy neighbour and watch Phil play catch or road hockey with his two sons. It uplifts me because Phil is a testimony to the fact that there is life post-transplant, and it is possible to run around and play with the kids like a normal, healthy person. As Phil, eight years post-transplant, put it, "I am thankful for restored health and the gift of everyday living. I think about the choice one family made to donate an organ, and I couldn't be more grateful. My life was saved because of organ donation, and because of that, I get the opportunity to enjoy watching my two amazing children grow up."

ABOUT THE AUTHOR

Christine Jowett is a registered cardiology nurse at St. Mary's Hospital. She enjoys being a nurse and helping patients with heart disease and plans on using her nursing background and experience as a transplant recipient to educate others on the importance of the gift of life.

Despite having written many essays and scientific reports for university, Christine never envisioned herself being a writer. However, when she was admitted to hospital for her liver transplant, she began to keep a journal in order to remember the details of her stay, what the doctors had told her, lab results, and so forth. Having continued to keep a journal during her post-op recovery, she was asked by her husband, family and close friends to write the story of her life.

Her transplant story was published in the Canadian wide newspaper "Hospital News" and in her hospital newsletter at St. Mary's General Hospital in Kitchener. However, it was her liver transplant on July 21, 2013 that led her to write this book, which is an emotional story based on a near death experience.

REFERENCES

Canadian Liver Foundation. "Autoimmune Hepatitis." http://www. liver.ca

National Institute of Diabetes and Digestive and Kidney Diseases. "Autoimmune Hepatitis." Last modified March 26, 2014. http://digestive.niddk.nih.gov/ddiseases/pubs/ autoimmunehep/#diagnosis

Wolters Kluwer Health. "Patient information: Autoimmune hepatitis (Beyond the Basics)." UpToDate. Last modified March 22, 2013. http://www.uptodate.com/contents/autoimmune-hepatitis-beyond-the-basics BeADonor.ca. http://www.beadonor.ca

Marino, Ignazio Roberto, Howard R. Doyle, Yoogoo Kang, Robert L. Kormos, and Thomas E. Starzl. "Multiple Organ Procurement." Accessed via University of Pittsburgh's D-Scholarship@Pitt. http://d-scholarship.pitt.edu/4996/1/31735062124817.pdf

Trillium Gift of Life Network. http://www.giftoflife.on.ca

Canadian Institute for Health Information. Tables re: 2011 organ donation and transplantation statistics for Canada. http://www.cihi.ca/CIHI-ext-portal/pdf/internet/ REPORT_STATS2011_PDF_EN

University Health Network. "Living Donor Liver Transplantation." Online manual forToronto General Hospital. http://www.uhn.ca/MOT/PatientsFamilies/Clinics_Tests/Documents/ LivingDonor_LiverDonorManual.pdf

University Health Network. "Post-Liver Transplant Manual." Toronto Liver Transplant Program. January 2012.

University Health Network. "Pre-Liver Transplant Manual." Toronto Liver TransplantProgram. 6th edition, January 2011.

Chan, Gabriel, Ali Taqi, Paul Marotta, Mark Levstik, Vivian McAlister, William Wall, and Douglas Quan. "Long-Term Outcomes of Emergency Liver Transplantation for Acute Liver Failure." *Liver Transplantation* 15 (2009): 1696-1702. DOI: 10.1002/lt.21931. Accessed via Wiley. http://onlinelibrary. wiley.com/doi/10.1002/lt.21931/pdf.

Finger, Erik B. "Organ Procurement Considerations in Trauma." Edited by Ernest Dunn, Francisco Talavera, Robert L. Sheridan, and John Geibel. WebMD Medscape. http://emedicine.medscape.com/article/434643-overview#aw2aab6b7

Norris, Sonya. "Background Paper: Organ Donation and Transplantation in Canada."

Library of Parliament (2011). http://www.parl.gc.ca/Content/LOP/ ResearchPublications/2011-113-e.pdf

University of Michigan Transplant Center. "How long can donated organ last outside thebody?" TransWeb.org FAQ. http://www.transweb.org/faq/q24.shtml

Feltracco, Paolo, Stefania Barbieri, Helmut Galligioni, Elisa Michieletto, Cristiana Carollo, and Carlo Ori. "Intensive care management of liver transplanted patients." World Journal of Hepatology 3, no. 3 (March 2011): 61-71. DOI: 10.4254/wjh.v3.i3.61. Accessed via PubMed. http://www.ncbi.nlm.nih.gov/pmc/articles/PMC3074087/#!po=48.0769

CONTACTS

Colleen Shelton
Manager, Multi-Organ Transplant Coordinator
University Health Network Toronto

Judy Wells
Organ and Tissue Donation Coordinator
for the Waterloo-Wellington area
Trillium Gift of Life